RAISING
VEGAN KIDS

RAISING
VEGAN KIDS

RAISING
VEGAN KIDS

LESSONS FOR LITTLES IN PLANT-BASED EATING
and
COMPASSIONATE LIVING

ERIC C. LINDSTROM
FOREWORD BY TESS CHALLIS

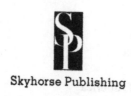

Skyhorse Publishing

Copyright © 2018, 2022 by Eric C. Lindstrom
Previously published as *The Smart Parent's Guide to Raising Vegan Kids* by Skyhorse Publishing in 2018.

All rights reserved. No part of this book may be reproduced in any manner without the express written consent of the publisher, except in the case of brief excerpts in critical reviews or articles. All inquiries should be addressed to Skyhorse Publishing, 307 West 36th Street, 11th Floor, New York, NY 10018.

Skyhorse Publishing books may be purchased in bulk at special discounts for sales promotion, corporate gifts, fund-raising, or educational purposes. Special editions can also be created to specifications. For details, contact the Special Sales Department, Skyhorse Publishing, 307 West 36th Street, 11th Floor, New York, NY 10018 or info@skyhorsepublishing.com.

Skyhorse® and Skyhorse Publishing® are registered trademarks of Skyhorse Publishing, Inc.®, a Delaware corporation.

Visit our website at www.skyhorsepublishing.com.

10 9 8 7 6 5 4 3 2 1

Library of Congress Cataloging-in-Publication Data is available on file.

Cover design by Eric C. Lindstrom and David Ter-Avanesyan
Cover photo credit by iStock

Print ISBN: 978-1-5107-6879-6
Ebook ISBN: 978-1-5107-7188-8

Printed in the United States of America

This book is dedicated to the
361,481 babies born each day
around the world.
May they all be raised vegan.

TABLE OF CONTENTS

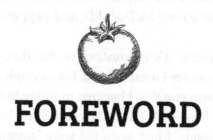

FOREWORD

You hold in your hands a book that will empower and inspire you to raise happy, healthy vegans. It can feel overwhelming to think about transitioning your family to a vegan diet, but Eric's down-to-earth (and fun) writing style will give you confidence and comfort.

As a vegan mom myself, Eric's book resonated with me on so many levels. For one thing, I love what he has to say about children being born compassionate (and vegan). I still remember my college days, working with children who often asked about my veganism. When I explained, quite simply, that I didn't eat animals or their products because it hurt them, they would almost invariably reply, "I want to be vegan, too!" (You guessed it—this usually didn't go over well with their parents when they found out.)

My daughter, now fifteen, has been vegan since birth, and although I haven't forced it on her, she's never wanted to stray. Perhaps this is why she's been a self-directed, dedicated vegan all her life—she simply needed the basic facts: that we thrive on plant-based foods, that animals suffer when we eat them, that dairy isn't healthy for humans, etc. I've encouraged her to think for herself, and just by doing that, veganism has *always* been the sensible, compassionate choice for her.

It doesn't hurt that her mom is a vegan cookbook author and cooking instructor, of course, but even in our household we have some challenges. In fact, Eric's book renewed my inspiration to take more control in the kitchen. My daughter's version of teenage rebellion means eating more vegan junk food and fewer veggies, which I don't love. However, there are things I can do to improve the situation, and ultimately, I'm just happy she's not eating McDonald's and pepperoni pizza like I did at her age.

Speaking of which, it's interesting to me that my daughter has avoided the health issues I used to have. For example, I had strep throat so many times growing up that I became immune to every antibiotic on the market. I also lived with constant headaches, low energy, anemia, and other health issues I just assumed were "normal." The fact that I grew up eating a Standard American Diet, and subsequently stopped having those health issues upon going vegan in 1991, is pretty telling. With her vegan diet, my daughter has yet to suffer from strep throat, and I can count the number of headaches she's ever had on one hand. Coincidence? Maybe, but I doubt it. Her vitamin levels have always been high, as have mine since going vegan.

It's also pretty cool that humans seem to have a natural preference for plant-based foods. (Hear me out!) If we're not conditioned to eat animal products, our taste buds prefer vegan food. I remember trying meat and dairy a few times after my first attempts to go vegan in 1990. The longer I ate a vegan diet, the less I enjoyed my old favorites. Eventually, foods I never thought I could give up (BBQ chicken and cheese sticks, for example) began to taste different—even disgusting—to me. My daughter has accidentally eaten animal products a few times, and she said the food tasted "gross" and didn't want to eat any more. Reverse that theory and give a nonvegan kid something vegan (such as an apple fritter or some potato pancakes) and you'll probably just get an enthusiastic request for seconds.

As Eric quotes from an anonymous speaker in the book, "Children are great imitators. So give them something great to imitate." So much of "teaching" our children actually boils down to being role models. More than listening to our words, children copy our actions. We don't need to be perfect, but as Eric's book suggests, let's strive to be examples of kindness, compassion, and healthy vegan eating. Part of why I can occasionally get my daughter to eat her veggies these days is because I eat mine. In fact, she often drinks a "Modified Mom," which is a less intense version of my kale-carrot-strawberry smoothie.

Can you get kids freakishly excited about healthy vegan food? Absolutely! I've found that with my own daughter, as well as with the hundreds of kids I've worked with over the years (most of whom weren't even vegetarian), it's all about delicious, fun food that leaves them feeling excited rather than deprived. You'd be amazed at how many meat-eating kids love vegan food! I vividly remember a young girl telling me, upon trying my recipe for "Raw Cinnamon Rolls," that her brain "suddenly turned on." Vegan foods are such a gift—for our planet, our bodies, and the animals.

So, if you're thinking about trying veganism—for yourself or your whole family—or you're already vegan and just need renewed inspiration, you'll find plenty in this book. Peruse the recipes, suggestions, and stories, and then go for it! And keep in mind, if a diehard foodie like me went vegan in 1991 (a year with zero decent vegan cheese on the market), you can do it in this vegan-friendly era! And always remember—you don't have to be perfect. You're already awesome for reading this book, so now go forth and be even more awesome, one bite at a time. You'll be so glad you did!

TESS CHALLIS
Author, vegan chef,
and "One Degree" coach

RAISING
VEGAN KIDS

RAISING
VEGAN KIDS

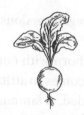

INTRODUCTION

"The future is always beginning now."
—*Anonymous*

So, you want to raise your kids vegan?

Well, good for you. Better for them. And most excellent for the planet and the animals.

Let me start right off by saying that this isn't going to be easy. Not so much the raising vegan kids part—this book is here to help with that, and I'll guide you, along with incredible insight from some of the leading plant-based thought leaders, through every step of the process. Now, combine going vegan with *parenting*? Well, let's say that kicks everything up a notch.

Parenting *is* the toughest job you'll ever encounter, and now add on that other layer of complexity by raising your kids to be compassionate vegans who won't eat (non-vegan) frosting straight from the container, who are concerned about the future of our shared planet, and won't consciously stomp on bugs.

I can't lie. My wife and I are raising two vegan kids ourselves, and it's a challenge. Raising your little ones without chicken nuggets, macaroni and cheese, and hot dogs—the usual kids' menu fare—takes commitment. Lucky for you, the parent who wishes to give your beloved offspring a jumpstart on excellent health and a compassionate attitude toward all living things, all of these same foods are readily available or are easy to make at home as vegan versions. Plus, have I mentioned that this book is here to help?

Every single one of us is born with compassion. Each of us begins life with a clean slate when it comes to attitudes and ideas about how all life on Earth should be regarded. A famous quote by Harvey Diamond, the best-selling author of the *Fit for Life* series of healthy dieting books, says "Put a baby in a crib with an apple and a rabbit. If it eats the rabbit and plays with the apple, I'll buy you a new car."

I'm willing to bet that Harvey hasn't had to buy anyone a new car. At least, I certainly hope not.

When confronted with the choice of eating an animal and not eating an animal, most infants and toddlers will choose *not* to eat an animal. Take any young child to a petting zoo, and nine out of ten of them aren't going to drool when they pet a pig or grope a goat. That tenth kid might need to be separated from the rest of the group. Actually, I'm pretty sure he should be separated—and you might also want to check on that kid groping a goat; something seems "off."

Over time, each one of us has been brainwashed by culture, tradition, and society to see meat, vis-à-vis animals, as food. To consume dead carcasses ourselves and then feed them to our children for three "balanced" meals a day has become so ingrained in our society that many kids aren't allowed to leave the table until they're done eating their cooked corpses. Punished for not wanting to dine on dead body parts.

"At least try a bite," my mom would say as I pushed around the small off-brown piece of veal on my plate with my fork. As a kid, and even as a meat-eating adult throughout the first half of my life—until I went vegan overnight on a bet—I never liked veal. Something about its texture felt like the afterthought of a good steak. Turns out, veal *is* an afterthought; a direct result of the dairy industry, in fact. The male offspring of dairy cows are most often destined for the veal crate (or studding or rodeo) since they, themselves, cannot become milking cows. So, they become meat.

Both outcomes—death before you turn the age of one or a lifetime of impregnation and lactation—are awful. Plus, veal, like most meats, has little to no actual taste. In fact, most meat only tastes good when prepared with spices, marinades, and sauces—all of which are made entirely of vegan-only ingredients.

Back to my mom's dinner table, I tried a bite. Choked it down. Was eventually allowed to leave to catch the second half of my and my little sister's favorite show, *Little House on the Prairie*. Turns out, they ate a lot of meat on the prairie. This is one of the main arguments of the proponents of meat-eating culture: we've always done it.

Eating meat, and the visuals associated with meat, have become a societal norm. They're everywhere. Vegans are often criticized for "pushing their agenda down everyone's throat," but TV, billboards, magazines, and 98 percent of restaurants are repeatedly pushing the omnivore's agenda 24/7. The earlier we can change perceptions about meat consumption and how it relates to animals, the easier it will be to successfully raise our kids vegan.

I can't tell you how many parents I know personally who struggle with the fact that their kids only eat certain foods. They complain that they can't get their kids to eat healthier or that their kids refuse to drink alt-milks.

"Xander is such a picky eater!" a well-intentioned parent said to me once, while we were perusing a buffet line at a local restaurant. "How do you get *your* kids to eat their vegetables?"

I really wanted to answer with, "Why'd you name your kid Xander?" But I didn't.

"Well, that's pretty much all our kids eat," I said. "Come to think of it, that's all they've ever eaten. I'd say that we 'got lucky,' but we have been committed from the start to make sure our kids eat healthy, plant-based foods. We're vegan."

Cue the judgmental look.

"Well, I could never get my Xander to eat broccoli," she huffed.

(I assume she has to say "my" Xander to separate him from the other Xanders. I took my kids to a museum recently and there were three Xanders within fifteen feet of each other. Not sure if they're planning some kind of coup, but that's *too* many Xanders in one place.)

"Blend steamed broccoli with some unsweetened non-dairy milk, toss in some raw cashews, fresh basil, and a little lemon," I said. "Add a pinch of salt, and you've just made a delicious broccoli pesto sauce. Serve it poured over his favorite pasta. He'll eat it."

And, just like that, Xander is now eating broccoli and has taken his first step toward becoming vegan.

I always like to remind these parents that they need to be clever (in more than just choosing baby names) and associate plant-based foods with the foods their kids already love. I also constantly remind them that *they're* the adult in the household.

Plus, this whole thing of raising a vegan kid will become more challenging as your kid grows older. Tweens and teens may have their own stubbornness when it comes to "traditional" dietary choices and may revolt at first. But I find there is a simple workaround. Until *they* get jobs that allow them to: 1) find a way to safely get to and from the grocery store; 2) make the purchase with their own hard-earned money; and 3) come home and make their own meals without burning down the house, *you're* still in charge of what's in the fridge and what goes onto their plates and into their bodies. They'll eventually eat what you make and will eventually not even know they're eating vegan (spaghetti with marinara as well as peanut butter and jelly are vegan).

Bear in mind that raising vegan kids is worth every ounce of the effort. There is nothing more rewarding than hearing your four-year-old ask for seconds of "dried out kale" or watching them scan a table of desserts and ask if the myriad of colorful cupcakes and cookies are vegan—before they finally decide to, happily, eat a piece of fresh fruit. In fact, there are no downsides of raising vegan kids.

Well, *maybe* one?

Sherry Colb, ethical vegan, Cornell law professor, parent of two vegan teens, and a close friend, considers that the only possible drawback of raising vegan kids is that it might arm their children with *something* to strike out with later on in their upbringing.

It could become the "thing" that a pre-pubescent might grab onto to revolt.

"I suppose when they decide to rebel against their parents that veganism may be a target," Colb commented when I asked if she felt there was any reason not to raise kids vegan. "At some point, it has to be *their* decision, and that might mean following the overwhelming majority of their peers and consuming a nonvegan diet. For vegan parents, this would be very disappointing. But that is not really a downside of being vegan as much as it is a downside of living in a nonvegan world. A lot of the inconveniences of veganism turn out to be just that—an inconvenience of having to find our way through a nonvegan society."

At the end of the day, you've hopefully had the time to reflect on what being vegan means to you and why you've chosen to raise your kids vegan. Is it for health, the planet, the animals, or all three? Veganism starts with food choices, no matter the reason, and the example you set will make the transition that much easier.

"As long as you're living under my roof!" takes on a whole new meaning when establishing a vegan household. As I've mentioned, since you control what's being purchased and what's being served, until your kids can fend for themselves (start with putting a bunny in their crib), they'll eat what you prepare. At least that's the idea. The Standard American Diet is S.A.D. Literally, sad. The food pyramid and the sources of nutrients and protein we've all been raised to believe are healthy exist entirely because of big money lobbyists, a struggling economy, and misinformation about nutrition—and it's literally killing us all. The very few fruits and vegetables we can usually get our kids to eat aren't the important leafy greens and the other superfoods that are packed with protein and essential nutrients.

Any guesses on what the number one vegetable consumed in the United States is? Potatoes. Translated to: French fries and potato chips. The number two vegetable? Iceberg lettuce, which is at the very bottom of the salad food chain. Its only "redeeming quality" is that it occasionally makes an appearance on fast food menus (primarily for photographic purposes), which allows it to sneak into little kids' diets atop a greasy burger, sandwiched between two buns.

The number three vegetable consumed in the United States is tomatoes, otherwise known as "where ketchup comes from."

French fries. Potato chips. Lettuce. And ketchup. Sound familiar?

Getting your kids to embrace being vegan and exploring a colorful world of amazing fruits and vegetables won't be simple, but soon they'll love "eating the rainbow." The phrase is more than just a platitude; the color of your food can say a lot about its nutritional value. Certain food colors indicate an abundance of specific nutrients—yellow and orange fruits and vegetables (for example, citrus fruits, varieties of squash) are abundant in vitamins C and A; green fruits and leafy-green veggies (kale, spinach, asparagus, avocado) are high in vitamins K, B, and E; purple produce (eggplant, red cabbage, grapes) are high in vitamins C and K.

The reason you can tell a food's nutritional value from their color is because plants derive their colors from various phytochemicals found in them.

phytochemicals [fi-to-kem-i-kuhs]
[noun] any of various bioactive chemical compounds found in plants, as antioxidants, considered to be beneficial to human health

Phytochemicals, as unappetizing as they may sound, are what offer the different nutrients in our food. In short, adding a variety of colorful produce to your kid's diet is an easy way to get a lot of vitamins and minerals without putting in too much effort. If your child eats ROYGBIV every day, you've pretty much got this whole vegan living thing figured out. Just remember "eat the rainbow." Which, by the way, is quite different from "Taste the rainbow," the tagline for the colorful candy Skittles. Although, amazingly, Skittles are actually on the ever-growing "accidentally vegan" list, as are Pop-Tarts, Doritos, Oreos, and Duncan Hines Double Fudge Decadent Brownie Mix.

You've got this.

Jamie Oliver, The Naked Chef and sometime FOV (Friend of Vegans), taped an episode of his show *Food Revolution* featuring a classroom full of young kids. Unbeknownst to them, they were about to be part of a fresh food experiment that would reveal that the majority—as in, all the kids—were unable to identify even the simplest fruits and vegetables. Oliver wanted to quiz these kids on the spot to see if they knew what fresh food looked like.

Oliver held up a vine-ripened bunch of tomatoes. "Who knows what this is?" The room goes dead silent, until a brave kid finally answered, "Potatoes?" The other kids were as perplexed by these red, round objects until Oliver asked, "Who knows what ketchup is?" All hands shot straight up, and it went downhill from there.

Our children are not connected to real, fresh, good food. You, as their parent, have a unique responsibility and opportunity to educate. Take them to the farmer's market or produce section of your local grocer. Let them learn the names, shapes, and smells of what they're going to eat.

Dr. Neal Barnard of the Physicians Committee for Responsible Medicine (PCRM), a not-for-profit in Washington, DC, that brings nutrition into medical education and practice, offers this advice to parents trying to introduce plant-based foods to their kids: "Children learn by example," he tells me. "Make sure you eat well in front of your child so that she perceives healthful eating as normal and worthy of emulating. Children naturally prefer simple foods—fruits, simple vegetables, grain products, and beans. Many children do not like meat when their well-meaning but ill-informed parents first introduce it."

Think about that. At some point growing up, you were most likely given an animal to eat, and this continued until you acquired a taste for eating them (as I've mentioned, animals only taste good because of the vegan spices and marinades used to prepare them). This is also how humans acquire their taste for dairy milk.

"You've probably heard it before, and that's because it works: keep reintroducing foods to your baby or child until she learns to like it," Barnard says. "They may push away the broccoli the first few times, but eventually, they'll try it . . . and like it!"

I have proof of this with my own two broccoli-gobbling little ones.

"Avoid power struggles," Barnard continues. "If your child doesn't like a certain food, don't force him or her to eat it."

Want more from Dr. Barnard and PCRM? Search for the incredible selection of papers and books written by him, and you'll discover he knows what he's talking about when it comes to healthy plant-based diets.

He also happens to be an amazing guitarist. Rock on, radish doctor. You've got the beet.

In 2016, the number of obese children and adolescents in the United States rose to 124 million—more than ten times higher than the 11 million classified as obese forty years earlier in 1975. Looking at the broader picture, this equated to almost 6 percent of girls and nearly 8 percent of boys who were obese just two years ago, and this trend shows no sign of slowing.

We owe it to our kids and their kids to get them on track with nutritious foods that won't continue this unhealthy trend—or strip the planet clean and dry.

As I've said, this book can help.

Raising Vegan Kids was written based on my own experience in going vegan (overnight); it is inspired by how my wife and I raised our two vegan toddlers; and it is mixed with professional insight, expertise, and knowledge from many other incredible plant-based practitioners, vegans, and animal rights activists.

Keep in mind that this book *will* focus a lot on diet and food choices, since that's the most challenging, and obviously first, step in going vegan. You'll be guided with expert advice from leading names in plant-based nutrition like Dr. Barnard, and find resources in the back of the book that will make ridding your house of all meat, dairy, and eggs as easy as possible. You'll also read accounts from parents of vegan kids, as well as from the vegan kids themselves.

But, just as important, you'll also learn about "the connection." That moment when it all comes together. When your choices on your dinner plate reflect your own ideals and philosophy on animal rights. Veganism is a lifestyle, not just a diet. In order to truly appreciate being vegan, you'll find yourself yearning to seek more information. You'll learn the "secret vegan handshake" one day and soon be able to watch your kids make their own kale smoothies (that can be easily modified to taste like a McDonald's Shamrock Shake, by the way).

This book will delve into veganizing your household and offer alternatives to some of the more popular baby and toddler necessities that can be vegan and cruelty-free. It will even help you help your dog transition to a vegan diet, since they are as much a part of the family as anyone else (it's not recommended that you make your cat vegan since they are natural carnivores and hunters). Our vegan dog, Kimchi, thrives on her diet and never has to think about whether the table scraps are healthy.

This book will also explore the entire universe and boldly go where no book has gone before. The future of our planet is at risk, and going vegan is one major step toward slowing and reversing some of the damage that has already been done. Animal agriculture has a greater carbon footprint on the planet than all the modes of transportation combined. As your family becomes vegan, you'll soon understand how your single drop in the ocean can become a massive wave toward your children's future and their children's future. Ride. This. Wave.

Finally, and arguably the most rewarding aspect of veganism of all, your kids will learn *compassion*. They will explore their emotional connections to *all* living beings. They will recognize the fact that this is a shared planet and that animals have as much a right to life as their companions. From the smallest spider that needs to finish spinning its web to the largest orca who belongs in the ocean and not in a tiny glass aquarium in San Diego—all living creatures deserve freedom and have a right to live.

Before I go much further, I want to mention that I recognize my privilege as a cis white heterosexual male living in the United States who is fortunate enough to have a steady income that allows me to afford certain luxuries, even simple ones like vegan cheese, that others may not. I am aware of this, and there may be parts of this book where this is more evident than others.

With that said, sit back, pour a cup of coffee (there are amazing vegan creamers on the market these days, by the way) and start your journey to veganism for your entire family. There is no time like the present.

Also, I know that "sitting back and pouring a cup of coffee" and starting *anything* is nearly impossible with kids around, so feel free to scan chapters quickly between changing diapers, breaking up fights, making dinner, patching wounded knees, patching holes in the wall, helping with homework, struggling to make dinner, or driving the kids to soccer practice. I've been there, and I *truly* appreciate all you do for your kids.

As I've mentioned before, this *won't* be easy.

But it *will* be worth it.

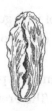

1

IN THE BEGINNING: BABIES, BOTTLES, AND BREASTS

"Animals are not products. Life doesn't have a price."
—*Anonymous*

ll babies are born vegan. In fact, they're vegan in the womb—if their biological mother is vegan. Food consumed by a pregnant mom travels down the food tube into the baby tube that connects to the fetal unit that nourishes the unborn child. This is all *very* technical, so please excuse the medical jargon. If you'd like me to draw up a supplementary illustration to show you how it all works, just ask.

In the womb, the fetus is fed the best of what's being put into the mom. A whole-foods, plant-based (vegan) diet transfers beautifully since it is so rich in vitamins, minerals, nutrients, and fiber (with no cholesterol and very little saturated fat). Up top, Mom can put as much vegan food into her body as she wants to help the growing, soon-to-be troublemaker become stronger and healthier, even prior to birth. Those hearty kicks after a bowl of quinoa salad with peanut lime dressing, followed by an almond milk peanut butter vanilla milkshake, will be a clear sign that eating right benefits both mom and baby.

(By the way, if you're vegan and pregnant and also happen to love kombucha, you may want to cut back on it until after the baby is born.

Even a small amount of alcohol isn't going to help your unborn baby's development. Cue a collective disappointed sigh from every pregnant woman in Portland.)

All that said, being pregnant is a perfect time to try *all* the vegan foods. The pizzas. The burgers. The French fries. The ice creams. Those incredible jackfruit tacos loaded with vegan sour cream and topped with shredded vegan cheddar cheese. Eat. All. The. Vegan. Foods.

Which is pretty much how I live my life now—and I'm not even pregnant.

Spend those nearly ten months nourishing your baby until they've had just about enough of that womb and are ready to take on the world, with unbridled compassion.

I remember when my youngest was born. Her mom ate a vegan diet and we, well before she was conceived, had planned to raise her and her brother 100 percent vegan. At the hospital, I looked into her eyes when she was just one minute old and six pounds and six ounces, so tiny and innocent and perfect, and I whispered to her, "You've got one hundred years to figure this all out." To which she replied with a strange duck noise that sounded just like, "Okay, Dad."

Wished I had recorded it, but you'll have to take my word for it.

I knew then what I know now, that with our help and the support of good people around her, she *is* going to thrive as a person, due, in part, to being raised vegan. In the hospital the following day, she latched onto her mother's breast and began her vegan lifestyle.

To lay to rest any ideas that breast milk isn't vegan, let me emphasize that breast milk *is* 100 percent vegan. Same species, with consent. Human breast milk is designed for human babies with their own nutritional needs and growth in mind. What about after the baby is weaned? Since cow's milk is designed for baby cows, it's not recommended for human babies (in spite of what countless pediatricians over countless decades have told you). In fact, cow's milk is as much intended for humans as dog, giraffe, chimpanzee, or dolphin milk. (By the way, did you know that dolphins actually nurse their offspring? How cute is that?)

The website BabyCenter.com, a worldwide pharmaceutical company owned by Johnson & Johnson, with a reach of more than 45 million parents *a month* from every corner of the globe through its eleven owned and operated online properties in nine different languages, says, "Babies can't digest cow's milk as completely or easily as breast milk or formula. Cow's milk contains high concentrations of protein and minerals, which can tax your baby's immature kidneys."

It continues: "Cow's milk doesn't have the right amounts of iron, vitamin C, and other nutrients for infants. It may even cause iron-deficiency anemia in some babies, since cow's milk protein can irritate the lining of the digestive system, leading to blood in the stools. Finally, cow's milk doesn't provide the healthiest types of fat for growing babies."

And, yet, somehow the very next paragraph under the above statement begins with: "However, once your child's *ready* to digest it . . ." It's almost as if feeding human babies the lactation from another species is wrong if they have to train their bodies to be able to digest it.

Allison Rivers Samson is a self-care coach, speaker, and workshop leader who helps women turn workouts into personal playdates, make healthy eating feel indulgent, and make room for themselves. She is also a parent to Olivia, a lifelong vegan, and she holds a certificate in plant-based nutrition from Cornell University. Allison is the cofounder of Dairy Detox and the author of the award-winning book *Veganize It!* She knows a thing or two about raising vegan kids.

I reached out to Allison to see if she had anything she wanted to say about nutrition and, specifically, dairy and breastfeeding. While I could have paraphrased her thoughts using my own perspective, I found her words to be so beautiful and moving that I've shared them as is:

My dairy-free life took on a whole new depth of meaning when I became a mother. It was a late afternoon, just a couple of short weeks after I'd given birth to my daughter. During one of our many nursing sessions, I looked down at her adorable little face, nestled in our shared warmth as she suckled my breast. A sudden mixture of sadness, protectiveness, and anguish crashed over me. I was confused and wondered how I could possibly feel mournful in this perfect moment.

And then it hit me—my sorrow wasn't for me and my baby; it was for a mother cow and hers. I got to hold my baby when she was still warm and wet, fresh from my womb, rather than having her dragged away shortly after birth to prevent bonding. I got to guide her to my breast and savor the sweetness of her warm little body close to mine as I nourished and nurtured her, instead of having the milk my body made for her be taken away and given to someone else. I got to be with her throughout her first vulnerable days, and I get to be with her now.

Even though cows and humans are different, cows have very strong maternal instincts just like humans do. Looking through the eyes of a cow, my experience of motherhood seems like a privilege. But it isn't. It is the birthright of every mother and child.

And yet, in the dairy industry, mothers and babies endure this heartbreaking loss over and over again throughout their unnaturally shortened lives. The exploitation these females and their babies are forced to suffer just to bring a chunk of cheese or a glass of milk to someone's table displays a depth of cruelty that's unimaginable to any human mother.

Is so much misery really worth a fleeting moment of pleasure on the palate, especially when there are so many other options that are even more delicious? No way. With a vast and growing number of delectable plant-based choices, we can easily choose both great taste and compassion in every bite.

So, when *do* you start your vegan baby on their vegan diet? And, if mom isn't vegan already, should she skip dairy products while breastfeeding?

"Start at conception," Dr. Neal Barnard says. "Seriously, there is no time during gestation, infancy, or any other time when children need animal products, except, of course, their mother's breast milk.

"Also, mom should follow a vegan diet while breastfeeding. Dairy proteins can pass from her digestive tract into her bloodstream and end up in her breast milk, and they can lead to colic and other problems in her baby."

Breast is best. Note: plant-based milk, as the packaging will warn you, is not a baby formula nor should it be considered a replacement for breast milk. And after your little one is weaned, the variety of nondairy milks on the mark today is absolutely astounding, and they are healthier than the healthiest cow's milk you'll find. Loaded with calcium, protein, vitamin D, and countless other vitamins and nutrients, they are the best first "food" following breastfeeding you could offer your infant. You can start your own little one on plant-based milks as early as age one, but keep in mind that it is a good idea to avoid nut-based milks, for possible allergies, and wait until they can talk. In our household, we have tried them all, and our two tiny toddlers drink up to three glasses a day. Note: tread lightly on nut milks in case your child has a nut allergy.

Almond milk: This is mostly what we drink interspersed between cartons of soy milk. To have your kids immediately fall in love with it, buy the sweetened vanilla variety. Tastes great on Fruity Pebbles (vegan) and Cheerios (also vegan). Sometimes, we will mix this with half soy milk to add more protein and to lower the sugar content.

Cashew milk: Creamier and thicker with more fat than most. I make homemade cashew milk as the base for vegan sauces and cheeses in our Vitamix with raw, soaked cashews. Simple soak your raw nuts (he he) for a couple of hours; then rinse, drain, and blend with water or a nondairy milk until creamy smooth. Add sweetener (dates or evaporated cane juice) for a sweet milk or garlic, salt, nutritional yeast, and lemon for an Alfredo sauce. By the way, I don't recommend bottle-feeding your infant Alfredo sauce; wait until they are a toddler.

Coconut milk: I think coconut milk tastes the most like its main ingredient. Not a bad thing if you love coconut and for when you're using it to make something sweet. It is most excellent when making Thai iced coffee or a piña colada cocktail. Of course, the latter is not recommended for anyone under the age of twenty-one.

Flax milk: Yep, they can make milk out of anything. Not one of our favorites, but probably one that's better for you than all the others in terms of nutrition. Each tablespoon of ground flaxseed contains about 1.8 grams of plant omega-3s.

Hazelnut milk: Unfortunately, I'm allergic and haven't tried it, but I've heard that many people love it (especially in their coffee).

Hemp milk: See? They use *everything*. I'm surprised there isn't a milk made out of peas (actually, see below). Hemp milk is actually really good and thick, and, like almond milk, it is much more enjoyable with the added vanilla flavoring.

Oat milk: Again, there's nothing like drinking something that's already proven healthy for you. A nondairy milk that helps your heart? Drink it up! Pour it on your Cheerios and *really* show love to your little one's ticker.

Pea milk: Maybe one of the first brands to come out with pea milk was Ripple, and it's delicious. Comes in a classic milk-jug-shaped packaging and is very thick and delicious. Pea protein is the new superfood that is making an appearance in countless vegan products.

Quinoa milk: Like flax milk, this one is loaded with all the goodness. Get your kids on any of these milks, and know that they're actually drinking something that will improve their health. Then, add chocolate—because you're a cool parent. PS Hershey's chocolate syrup is vegan.

Rice milk: This was the first nondairy milk I tried, and I still think it is the closest to taste and appearance to cow's milk. There's not a ton of nutritional value, but with all the fortification (B12, vitamin D, vitamin E, and calcium) they add, it's still better for you than cow's milk.

Soy milk: This is probably the most well-known and most "controversial" of the nondairy milks, since the meat and dairy industries want you to believe that soy is bad for you. It's not. It's a bean. It would be like avoiding chickpea milk, which by the way, they just came out with.

With alt-milks, along with the rainbow of colorful fruits and vegetables and hearty grains, you'll soon be spoon-feeding your precious peanut and setting them up for a lifetime of great health. Pro tip: get a high-speed blender like a Vitamix or Blendtec. They are perfect for everything—from making your own plant-based milks and baby foods to delicious smoothies and the creamy Alfredo sauce I just mentioned. We use ours at least once a day.

Know someone whose kid is lactose intolerant? Well, technically, they're not actually lactose-intolerant; they're just not calves. The son of one of our friends is "lactose-intolerant," and instead of any of these amazing, delicious plant-based milks listed above, they are giving him goat's milk.

To be fair, goat's milk is naturally lactose-free. However, goats suffer in the same way as cows in regard to milk production for humans. Cow's milk is for calves, and goat's milk is for kids (by *kid*, I'm referring to the name by which we call baby goats). Gorilla milk is for gorillas, and human milk is for humans.

And that image of nursing dolphins is still adorable.

2
MILK: IT DOES A BODY BAD

"Life is too short to make others' shorter."
—*Anonymous*

More on milk?
Dairy, which includes milk and cheese, may be the most difficult thing to eliminate when going vegan and possibly the most misunderstood by new parents. So, I've decided to dedicate a good portion of the beginning of this book to it. Adults already struggle with giving up dairy, and getting kids on board is equally challenging. In fact, a study published in *PLOS One* proved that the number one most difficult food to give up, over every other food, is pizza.

Because?

Well, first of all, it's pizza, the single greatest food ever invented.

pizza [peet-suh]
[noun] a flat, open-faced baked pie of Italian origin, consisting of a thin layer of bread dough topped with spiced tomato sauce and cheese. The single greatest food ever invented.

All of that delicious grease, salt, and . . . opiates.

"Papa John's! How can I help you?" The pimply-faced boy cheerfully chirped into the phone with as much authority as he could muster. The pimples are assumed.

"I'd like a large pizza, extra cheese, and extras opiates, please. Oh, and extra garlic dipping sauce," I said. This would have been my pre-vegan order (though the dipping sauce happens to be vegan).

"Let me see if I got this right: large pizza, extra cheese, extra opiates, and extra garlic dipping sauce?" He cracked, like Peter Brady.

"That's it."

"That'll be eleven dollars and ready in twenty minutes."

Mmmm opiates. Scientifically speaking, cheese is as addictive as morphine, and the more "cheesy" something is, the harder it is to quit. So, while pizza may top the list of foods that are tough to surrender, ice cream is also in the top five and other milk-containing foods (like milk chocolate) are all over the top ten.

Milk is not easy to quit.

From a glass of cold milk and thick Greek yogurt to creamy ice cream and melty cheese, so many favorite foods are made from milk or contain milk. However, said that being said, it *is* the single most important animal byproduct to eliminate from your family's diet. Two of the foremost authorities on the dangers of milk in a person's diet today are Drs. T. Colin Campbell and Thomas M. Campbell, co-authors of the best-selling book *The China Study* who have written volumes on the health dangers of milk. T. Colin Campbell once told me personally that he thinks milk is more important to remove from your diet than even meat for health reasons. (Still, remove meat.) We've been fed the myth that humans need milk for calcium, even while clinical research shows that calcium in dairy products have little or no benefit for bones. People often drink milk in order to obtain vitamin D in their diets, unaware that they can receive vitamin D through other sources (including a ten-minute walk outside during daylight). Actually, few foods naturally contain vitamin D, and *no dairy products naturally* contain this vitamin. Fortified cereals, grains, bread, orange juice, and soy or rice milk are excellent options for providing vitamin D through diet, as are mushrooms, which happen to be my favorite pizza topping.

Amazingly, consumption of dairy products has also been linked to higher risk for various cancers, especially cancers of the reproductive system—prostate, ovarian, and breast cancers. In fact, Dr. T. Colin Campbell calls casein, the animal protein found only in milk, the number one fuel for the cancer fire.

And what about pesticides? Polychlorinated biphenyls (PCBs) and dioxins are examples of contaminants found in milk. According to Dr. Campbell, dairy products contribute about one-fourth to one-half of our dietary intake of total dioxins, and these toxins do not readily leave the body and can eventually build to harmful levels that may affect the immune, reproductive, and central nervous systems. Moreover, these PCBs and dioxins have *also* been linked to cancer.

Milk proteins, milk sugar, fat, and saturated fat in dairy products pose health risks and encourage the development of obesity, diabetes, and heart disease—in children. So, why are parents so set on introducing dairy to their bright-eyed, freshly-weaned infants?

When preparing to write this book, I went straight to Dr. Tom Campbell, who happens to be a friend of mine and the father of a vegan toddler and a newborn. "How bad *is* milk for humans?" I asked. "And how are you sure *your* kids are getting enough nutrition without it?"

"Pediatricians have been taught that dairy is essential," Campbell said. "It's in all the standard pediatrics histories that we learn to go over with parents. Oftentimes, the standard American kid diet is loaded with cheese. Lots and lots of cheese, several times a day, with snacks of yogurt and milk over sugar cereal. In this case, dairy would be a great target number one [to eliminate].

"Whole-food, plant-based diets are richer in most, but not all, nutrients. Having looked at this question in detail, I feel confident about this. We supplement our older kid, who is weaned, with B12 and vitamin D, and occasionally iodine (we don't eat many sea vegetables, which are rich in iodine). Our newborn is exclusively breastfed, and my wife supplements with B12 and D and occasionally some iodine.

"Apart from the number crunching aspect of having looked at the nutrient content of a well-planned plant-based diet, we also know that our kids are growing and developing well, which is reassuring. In general, this is the way most physicians assess whether a kid is getting enough calories and nutrients in general: growth and development."

Years ago, I had a friend whose physical therapist told her to cut out dairy as it was possibly the cause of her back pain. Back then, during my omnivorous days, I refused to believe that milk could be bad for your bones (and that I would ever take something like milk away from my kid). I was one of the millions of people who have been lied to about the health benefits of dairy. Years later, as a vegan, I actually met her physical therapist. I retold this story to her and found out that my friend's back pain has since completely gone away since giving up dairy.

A recent study, published in the *British Medical Journal*, examined milk intake and its relationship to risk of bone fractures, death from "any cause," and death from cardiovascular disease and cancer in a large group of Swedish men and women. Contrary to what you might expect, among middle-aged and older women, each additional glass of milk consumed daily was associated with a 9 percent increased risk of hip fracture and a 15 percent increased risk of death from any cause. Adding an extra glass of milk was also associated with a 15 percent increased risk of death from heart disease.

This is why your own grandmother or grandfather has fallen and can't get up. Since they were a little child, they were told that milk was helping with their bone density when, in fact, the opposite was taking place.

While dairy has been a part of our diet since humans first figured out how to milk a cow, it's really been since World War I that the industry itself, now armed with a nine-billion-dollar advertising budget per year, became the powerful force it is today.

Back in the day, there was a dairy surplus. The USDA Dairy Division began to advertise the benefits of cow's milk by developing educational milk campaigns that were rolled out nationwide to move the milk and assist dairy farmers in staying profitable. World War I ended a hundred years ago, and they're still trying to keep the outdated industry afloat. Needless to say, through these early efforts, they were successful in their goal to increase demand. Between the first and second world wars, advertisements for dairy linked milk consumption to bone health, calcium, and vitamin D, and mothers across America started to increase dairy intake in their households. Soon, even doctors were on board believing the myth.

Dairy marketing continues today at an even more fervent pace, from posters in the school cafeterias to outdoor advertising in every major city in the country. The message is always something along the lines of: "Milk will make you strong, and the protein and calcium in milk are a required part of a balanced diet."

The dairy industry recently waged a direct attack on the alt-milk industry. Targeting an ever-growing popularity of plant-based milks, they released messages like "Real milk isn't made from beans and nuts" and "Real milk requires no shaking." The campaign by the Irish Dairy Industry even stated that their milk was truly "plant-based," since their cows eat plants.

The battle rages on between those who know the truth and those who live the myth. With your kids, you have a unique opportunity to change the conversation, *now*. When you start a habit young, like going vegan, it's more likely to be a habit for life.

Curriculum for seventh and eighth graders from the National Dairy Council (NDC) promoted milk and other dairy products as the single best sources of calcium, stressing to children that fruits and vegetables just aren't enough. Look at any food diagram sent to schools or "healthy-eating" plates, and you'll see that they all stress the importance of milk in a healthy diet. Harvard University noted that even with a high intake of calcium, your risk of osteoporosis (bone disease) may not even be lowered. More isn't always better, which is why the nutrition community calculates both lower and upper limits for recommended nutrient intakes—including dairy. Add to this the number of people in this country who are "lactose intolerant" (i.e., "not baby cows"), and you soon realize that milk may not be what we've been told it is. In the United States, about 25 percent of all people lose their ability to break down lactose after weaning; and this number increases to 75 percent worldwide.

Even when a food is high in certain nutrients, this does not mean the nutrients will be easily absorbed by our bodies; it hinges somewhat on the makeup of the food as a whole. For instance, spinach and chard are not optimal sources of calcium because they contain oxalic acid, a compound that prevents the absorption of calcium. Not to worry, vegans and lactose-intolerant folks alike: calcium is easily absorbed from kale, collards, mustard greens, turnip greens, bok choy, broccoli, fortified plant milks, fortified juices, and firm tofu made with calcium-sulfate. You can get all the calcium you need without drinking a single glass of milk.

A single serving of the soy milk we have in our fridge at the moment provides 45 percent of the USRDA (United States recommended daily allowance) of calcium—as well as 16 percent protein, 100 percent Vitamin B12, and 30 percent Vitamin D—needed for a healthy diet. Two glasses of this per day, along with regular plant-based meals, and your littles are fully fortified to take on the world—while saving the planet and the animals. Keep in mind that this can also be poured over a nutritious breakfast cereal or turned into a delicious smoothie or banana shake.

Meanwhile, it turns out that the protein in cow's milk (and in all animal products) appears to actually *acidify* the blood. One of the body's main priorities is to keep our blood at a neutral pH. To buffer the acid in our blood, our bones release calcium. So, drinking milk to get calcium seems a little bit counterproductive. This phenomenon may explain why countries with high milk consumption have high rates of osteoporosis, while countries with low milk intakes don't seem to have problems with bone fractures. Yet, pediatricians still recommend cow's milk, and parents still feed it to their offspring.

All this goes to show that money is power. The dairy industry spends a significant amount of money on lobbying—nearly a billion dollars a year—by infiltrating schools and reaching youth with their products and "educational materials," using medical professionals to advocate for them, running manipulative advertising campaigns that play on our fears (and are paid for by our tax dollars, by the way), and influencing the government's dietary guidelines. The dairy industry is shaping our food environment and the messages we receive about cow's milk, which has certainly influenced our food choices.

Today, the dairy lobby still continues using tactics to keep the calcium/health myth alive. You *can* get all the calcium and nutrients you need from plants, without supporting the cruelty of the dairy industry and consuming health-threatening animal protein, bad cholesterol, blood and pus, or saturated fat. Plant-based milks and nondairy milk products are delicious and nutritious and can easily become a part of your family's regular diet.

Start here. Get your kids to love plant-based milk, yogurt, ice cream, and cheese first. The rest of the foods will fall into place after that. In fact, once you start them off early, they will not only never miss drinking cow's milk but will also find the flavor offensive compared to what they're drinking.

Milk comes from a cow. But not any ordinary cow; This cow has to be lactating. And, as we all know, in order to be lactating, you have to have recently given birth.

Parents, you may want to cover your little one's ears for this next part.

In order to have given birth, the cow has to be pregnant. And, as we all know, the easiest way to impregnate a cow is to insert your arm far into the cow's rectum in order to position the uterus and then force an instrument into the cow's vagina to artificially inseminate her. The restraining apparatus used is commonly called a "rape rack," and it's not a very pleasant image or experience for the animal.

Once pregnant, the cow waits about the same amount of time as a female human to give birth. The big difference is that once she gives birth, her newborn calf is forcibly taken from her so milk drinkers can get the milk they want for their bowl of Frosted Flakes.

If the newborn is female, she will likely be raised to live the same life as her mother—subjected to a life of servitude and imprisonment while constantly being impregnated to keep her milk flowing. If the newborn is male, well, that lucky little feller will be kept lucid in a small plastic box and killed within the first few months of his life for veal or sent off to rodeo. The lucky ones are sent to stud, which also isn't as glamourous as it sounds.

Now that she's rid of her pesky calf, this old girl is ready for a-milking!

Ah, the romance of milking a cow. You might conjure up the image of a farmer firmly grabbing hold of the cow's teats, rolling down his fingers, and pulling on each nipple until milk begins to squirt out and fill his bucket. The truth is, in nearly every instance around the world, the cow is instead hooked up to a painful milking apparatus that automatically milks her for hours on end, leaving her bloodied and sore to the point where infection causes pus and blood to get mixed with the milk, which in turn becomes part of the decadent bowl of ice cream you *used* to enjoy.

Once the cow stops producing milk, the cycle begins all over again until the cow reaches a point where she can no longer get pregnant—and then she's killed.

This is the dairy industry.

If you're already vegan and trying to raise your kids vegan, eliminating dairy is behind you, and you're not a part of this process. Thank you. But if you're starting fresh and are wondering where to begin, dump the dairy.

Getting rid of milk in your family's diet is like eliminating glue in your toddler's tummy. According to a study conducted by Dr. Michael Greger and NutritionFacts.org, dairy is the leading cause of chronic constipation in children; an immune response to cow's-milk protein has been proposed as a possible cause. I can't tell you how many play-dates have been cancelled by other parents because their little one is stuck on the potty.

Cow's milk is extremely hard on everyone's digestive system, especially children's. Consider this: cows have four stomachs. Last time I checked, kids only have one. Plus, pasteurization kills all the probiotics in milk that would help with digestion if the milk were left raw (which may be one reason why some people drink raw milk, which grosses me out to no end). Amazingly, the elimination of all dairy products was found to cure constipation in up to *100 percent* of kids, according to the same study.

Drinking cow's milk is utter nonsense.

Take it from someone who recently had two in diapers: vegan kids don't get constipated. In fact, whatever the opposite of constipation is, that's what my kids have. They have a minimum of two healthy poos per day, and sometimes they decide to poo in unison. I couldn't be more proud.

What causes the dramatic increase in bowel movements for vegans? In one word—fiber. So many of us in the western world are fiber deficient, and many experts believe it to be one of the biggest public health problems facing us today.

Perfect poops aside, what other immediate benefits can your offspring expect in their future now that they're being raised on a milk-free, vegan diet?

- Possible elimination of asthma
- No more eczema or acne
- Reduced risk of heart disease
- Less likely to get cancer
- Better hair, nails, and skin
- Increased energy levels (this could explain my boy)
- Reduced occurrences of allergies

And, knowing that they're saving thousands of lives.

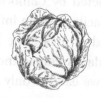

3
BORN COMPASSIONATE:
BITE AN APPLE/PET A BUNNY

"Animals are here with us, not for us."
—Anonymous

Most children do not want to eat animals at an early age; they usually have to be *forced* to eat them. Eating animals is not instinctual. Think about it; it is the same as admitting that your kid salivates while playing with goats at a petting zoo. Humans are not natural carnivores.

"Now, Emma, don't bite that goat. How many times do I have to tell you? Emma! Off. That. Goat." Emma, like the other 74 million children under the age of eighteen in the United States, doesn't have an instinctual appetite for goat, chicken, cow, or pig—that is, until she has been trained to eat it. Animals are not a natural human food.

When you teach your children to demonstrate compassion toward all living things and allow them to separate sentient beings from their dinner plates, I promise that you'll see them full of joy. They're happier, they're friendlier. You also most likely won't see them bullying other kids on the playground.

We've seen this in our own infant from a very young age, and it has also been proven in the prison-industrial complex (stay with me).

An experiment was conducted by California's Victor Valley Medium Community Correctional Facility, where inmates were offered a plant-based menu option instead of meat. The facility's nutrition services coordinator, Julianne Aranda, explained their main reason for offering a plant-based diet, "What we eat not only affects us physically, but it affects our mental attitude, our aggressiveness, and our ability to make good decisions."

When the facility launched the program, they didn't expect too many inmates to want to get involved. But as it turned out, a whopping 85 percent signed up. And as many as 95 percent of those who were introduced to a vegan diet have stayed vegan since taking part in the program. Furthermore, over time, the number of violent incidents actually decreased. The administration at the facility mentioned that there was a noticeable difference in the personalities of the vegan inmates. They smiled more, were fully racially integrated, and attended religious classes and anger management classes eagerly. Within just ten days, the vegan inmates expressed improvement in how they felt. They were not only feeling great from a physical standpoint; they also felt great from a standpoint of compassion.

Then, the Federal Bureau of Prisons introduced its new national menu for the 2017 fiscal year—which included Tofu Fried Rice, Soy Taco Salad, Bean Burritos, and Soy Hot Dogs—and says the unprecedented move came after an annual assessment of inmate eating preferences and other operational factors. "The Bureau seeks to provide a variety of options, including vegan options, which also support religious dietary accommodations," Justin Long, spokesperson for the Federal Bureau of Prisons, said. Earlier that year, actress and long-time animal rights activist Pamela Anderson made headlines when she urged the Louisiana prison system to adopt a vegan menu in an effort to save taxpayer money, promote healthier eating, and spare animal lives.

Veganism has shown that it brings about positive changes in people young and old.

Speaking from experience, I can say that raising kids vegan is simply the best way to raise children—with empathy and compassion for everything. We need to teach our children about the things we have done wrong (we must admit our faults) and try to change our societal thinking to one where we care for everything. Where we understand that the planet *doesn't* just exist for humans. Where other animals have as much a right to their freedom as we do, and in taking care of them, we become the voice for the voiceless. It's important to teach children compassion, which goes hand-in-hand with veganism.

Good at crocheting? Crochet the word *Ahimsa* and point this out to your kids every morning over their bowl of Cap'n Crunch's Peanut Butter Crunch cereal (yes, vegan) drenched in vanilla almond milk.

Ahimsa [əˈhimˌsä/]
[noun] (in the Hindu, Buddhist, and Jain tradition) the principle of nonviolence toward all living things

It's really very simple, obvious, and black and white to kids. Encouraging them to be inquisitive and to not be afraid to ask questions opens up a whole floodgate of conversations that can help them nurture empathy and a deeper understanding of the idea of a shared planet.

If your kid currently isn't vegan, ask them why they eat animals and listen to their answer.

In our household, we constantly remind our little ones that animals are not food. We encourage them to talk to us about what they are eating, and they're always the first to mention to other friends and family members that they don't eat animals. They go so far as to point out on other friend's plates the foods that are vegan and the foods that aren't.

Our job as parents, and ambassadors for planet Earth, is to keep the world in balance and to protect it. We simply have to encourage this dialogue and conversation, and our kids are going to take it from there.

Sherry Colb has had her own experiences raising her two vegan kids, Meena and Amelia.

"We have never found it difficult to deal with our friends or our children's friends when it comes to veganism," she said. "People have been largely accepting, though they occasionally ask questions (and we can now direct them to *Mind If I Order the Cheeseburger?* when they ask those questions)."

Sherry's book, *Mind If I Order the Cheeseburger?*, covers nearly every conceivable question encountered by a vegan. She answers them in escalating levels of detail until you're finally left with nothing but the absolute truth, stripped of opinion, to contemplate. By the end of the book, Sherry shows how it's possible for vegans and nonvegans to engage in a mutually beneficial conversation, without descending into counterproductive name-calling, and to work together to create a more hospitable world for human animals and nonhuman animals alike. With each answer, Sherry, who is a professor of law, rests her case.

"I recall one neighbor whose children played with Amelia. Amelia asked the mom why she eats nonvegan food. The woman thought for a moment and then replied, 'Because I'm not vegan.' She smiled as though she had given a very clever response. That was no answer at all, however; a bit like responding to the question 'Why do you kill animals?' with 'Because I kill animals,' but the woman did not seem to realize this. She wasn't hostile, though. As a general matter, we do not explicitly try to recruit our friends to veganism, but quite a few of them have come to veganism on their own, and we like to think that our way of living inspired them. We know that our kids have inspired other children to try or commit to veganism."

As well as grown men. As it turns out, Sherry's older daughter, Meena, can take full responsibility for me becoming vegan. And not just from a dietary perspective, which is where it started for me, but eventually from an ethical perspective too—being vegan for the animals.

I was officially challenged to go vegan at the end of 2011. It was Meena who approached me when she was just eight years old and suggested that Jen, my wife, and I should go vegan. At that point in my life, veganism was the furthest thing from my mind. I was a notorious meat-eater and would only eat vegetables if they were dipped in something—or if I was being forced. Meena planted the seed during a whole-foods, plant-based dinner that later turned into a bet that grew into a lifestyle that became a blog that became a book. In 2017, six years later, I published *The Skeptical Vegan.*

But back to the beginning, Meena's suggestion led my wife, Jen, to buy the book *The 30-Day Vegan Challenge* by Colleen Patrick-Goudreau. Colleen is a cultural commentator, bestselling author, and someone I am fortunate enough to call a friend today. She was there for me at the start of my very own vegan journey, with words of wisdom; and she is there for me today as I write my (second) book, sharing insights and inspiration we can all learn from about raising vegan kids. She tells me:

Like most children, I cared deeply for animals and intervened whenever they needed aid. My affection for and connection with animals was fostered by my parents and the adults around me—I was dressed in clothing that featured images of baby animals; I had stuffed animals all over my bedroom; I sang songs, read books, watched movies, and played games that used animals not only to teach me how to be polite, generous, and kind, but, even more significantly, how to read, how to spell, and how to count. I was the child who saved injured birds, sheltered stray animals, and stayed up whole nights comforting my dog when she was a scared puppy or sick adult. My parents commended me for demonstrating such kindness, and I was called an "animal-lover," as are so many of us who share an affinity for animals, but I don't think it is necessarily a fitting moniker. I don't believe you have to love animals in order to not want to hurt them.

And yet, I was hurting them. I was eating them.

I grew up being fed the typical American fare: turkey sandwiches, ice cream, and hamburgers. I didn't choose these foods. They were chosen for me. Nobody told me what they were made from, and when I asked, my parents either evaded the question entirely or deceived me completely. Early on, I learned that animals were arbitrarily categorized in our society: those worthy of our compassion and those undeserving of it because they happen to be of a particular species or bred for a particular use. Puppies, good. Calves, food.

As a child, I was taught that my dog was worthy of love and affection, but the animals whose dismembered bodies covered my dinner plate—and who are as capable of feeling pain and fear as any dog, cat, or human—were worthless. I was taught that the injured bird who was lucky enough to fall into my yard was worth saving, but the chickens and turkeys who I was deceptively told 'gave their lives for me' were valuable only in so far as their flesh was tender and juicy. Chickadees, friends. Chickens, dinner.

The consequences of this socially sanctioned cognitive dissonance are certainly grave for the victims of our appetites, but I would argue that they're equally grave for us. Going from innately compassionate children who identify deeply with animals to desensitized adults who justify our violence against them cannot but affect us at the most basic level—both individually and as a society. In fact, empathy for and kindness toward animals is one of the barometers we use to measure the emotional and mental health of both children and adults, and we're justifiably concerned when someone is overtly unkind to—or derives pleasure from harming—an animal, and we shield children from participating in or witnessing animal suffering because we are aware of the trauma it causes, both to the victim as well as the onlooker. And yet, we support it nonetheless.

There is a school of thought that says people who raise their children vegan are imposing their values on them and taking away their choice. Balderdash! Parents impose their values on their children all the time. It's called parenting. As an adult, I had to undo all of the conditioning I had been raised with, because I was told one thing ("be kind") but taught the opposite ("eat animals"). When I discovered what had been hidden from me, I woke up—literally. It was like a veil was lifted from my eyes and my heart, and I stopped eating animals, their eggs, and milk. I "became vegan." Having been conditioned to suppress my compassion for animals, it was liberating to have my actions reflect my values of nonviolence, simplicity, and kindness. Ignorance is indeed bliss—for only those who aren't the victims.

It was only when I was willing to look at how I contributed to violence against animals that I became awake, and in doing so, I have not so much returned to the innocent compassion of my childhood but instead have found a deeper place—where my eyes and heart are open not because of what I don't know but because of what I do know.

May we create for ourselves and for the children of our world a legacy of unabashed, unconditional, unrestrained compassion, and may we teach them the value of consistently manifesting their deepest values in their daily behavior.

On January 4, 2012, I was eating whatever I wanted and washing it down with whatever I could find; on January 5, the next day, I woke up 100 percent vegan with Colleen's book by my bed. I pretty much went to bed with chicken wing sauce on my fingers and woke up pressing tofu. In fact, my whole vegan saga is the subject of the book *The Skeptical Vegan* (Skyhorse Publishing), available wherever fine books are sold.

I was the last person on the planet you'd ever expect to go vegan. Jen was a gluten-free vegetarian in denial about being lactose intolerant, and I was a known omnivore with definite leanings toward carnivore. If it wasn't beef, it was chicken. If it wasn't chicken, it was pork. Once a year, it was turkey. On Friday, it was fish. I ate shark, octopus, conch, lamb, goat, deer, duck, goose, squirrel, bison, and even bear. If it can be killed, butchered, baked, or barbecued, there is a very good chance I've eaten it at one point in my life. For the record, and in case this book winds up in the hands of the FBI, I've never eaten an eagle—at least not a bald one.

I was having a lifelong love affair with meat, and we were never breaking up.

Then, one day, there I was—vegan. It wasn't easy at first. In fact, I was very reluctant and, well, skeptical. The least of my worries was "where would I get my protein" when all I could worry about was when would I get to eat chicken wings again.

Obviously, I'm still vegan today, as is Jen, our two toddlers, and the dog. And, looking back, I've shared many of the early challenges and the same questions that you, too, may have faced or are about to face as you raise your own kids vegan:

Why Are There No Vegan Options?

I'll never forget after first going vegan how adamantly I expressed to all my newfound vegan friends that there are "no good options" for eating vegan on-the-go—this phenomenon was clearly displayed in any vending machine in any bus or gas station in America. I was very sure of myself when I mentioned all the food a vegan could not buy while traveling.

Luckily, on-the-go vegan food does exist and there is a comprehensive list at the back of this book (page 142). Today, vegan options are popping up everywhere and the quality is improving at an incredible rate. In fact, anything I used to eat as an omnivore now has a vegan (and healthier) option.

However, please note that you should not be feeding your kids food from vending machines in the first place. It is not good for you and definitely not a good example to set for your littles.

And I bet you didn't know that *every* grocery store in America has a full vegan section. It's called "produce."

Will Your Health Actually Improve?

When I first went vegan, I was very skeptical about the health advantages, assuming that losing protein, B12, D-whatever, and all the amazing health benefits of eggs would turn me into a scrawny weakling. Of course, within the first six months, the exact opposite happened. I did, in fact, lose weight (a total of thirty pounds in the first year) and soon discovered that my energy level increased, my hair was thicker, my skin was clearer, and ... well ... I was pleased to also discover the incredible benefits of veganism in bed (and I'm not talking about sleeping; this is why we have a second vegan infant).

It was within the first two years that I really started to pay attention to what I was eating and exploring new foods that fueled my new vegan body. I learned from many of the leading experts in whole-foods, plant-based nutrition (through conferences and documentaries, many of whom are quoted in this book) and can now go toe-to-toe with any omnivore when talking nutrition.

Where Will I Find Vegan Support?

Soon after going vegan, I realized I was going to lose a few friends. The friends with whom I used to sit around a campfire eating fresh-caught fish or the gang who would get together over a chicken wing special. If there is one downside to going vegan for me, this is probably it. But it happens when you make any radical lifestyle change, and I learned to accept it.

Of course, the upside is that you get to meet and make new friends. Starting with local meetups and vegan clubs and joining every vegan Facebook group of interest, within a couple years I built an entire peace-loving army of vegans whom I consider my friends. Getting together with them is every bit as rewarding, if not more, as with my original group.

Plus, those old omnivore buddies will go vegan one day . . . everyone will.

Would I Be Able to Go the Distance?

Probably the thing that made me most skeptical about going vegan was whether or not it would last. Whether or not I would be able to go the distance. Would I fold or cheat or make excuses? For example, I know someone who has a 100 percent vegan diet except for cream cheese.

It was within the first year that I knew I was forever vegan, and this is the one thing I tell anyone who is considering a vegan lifestyle for your family: once you've made the connection, there is no going back. Once you've connected the dots and understood that animals deserve to live and that their byproducts are not ours to consume, you will be forever vegan.

I can remember staring at a field of grazing cows when I made this connection. I pulled my car over and watched them as they went on with their morning. Enjoying the sunshine. Eating whatever it is they eat. Bumping into each other. Frolicking. Loving. Living.

These animals, who bond with each other and treat each other like family, had as much a right to live as I did. Once I had this epiphany, I knew I was vegan for life.

For their lives.

Am I Actually Saving the Planet?

I was also skeptical about my own impact on the planet. Would cutting meat, dairy, and eggs really reverse global warming and protect the polar bears? How could my food choices have any effect on the future of our planet?

They do. Every choice I make helps. Every choice *you* make helps. Plus, my voice has become loud about veganism and the fragility of planet Earth. While I know my own choices are already making a difference, more important, I know that the hundreds of people I've educated over the past five years will make an even bigger impact.

I am but one who can change many.

So, how does raising vegan kids make a difference? They are the future. If you're compassionate—and passionate—enough, seeing them thrive as vegans will silence some of the initial fears you may have. If you get started on your and *their* journey, and see it through, it will grow into something amazing.

After I survived the initial thirty days as a vegan, I decided to make the challenge more interesting. I took it up a notch and placed a wager with my wife in the beginning of January. The Bet. The first to break would have to do chores for three months while the other watched. Seeing as how Jen was addicted to cheese, I was confident that I would both win the bet *as well as* go back to my meat-eating, milk-drinking, egg-cracking ways by the end of February. I'd be sitting back eating meatloaf and gravy while I watched her vacuum and dust.

Now, almost seven years and two books later, I'm still vegan. It's still the bet I refuse to lose, and now our entire family is vegan. And we're responsible for encouraging and supporting countless new vegans as they navigate their own path.

My diet in the beginning consisted of beans and nuts and lettuce and rice. And more beans and rice. Pretty much a list of all the foods I used to avoid. It was difficult staying true to the vegan lifestyle in the first few weeks, but I refused to give in and I persevered.

Two weeks after the bet, while on a business trip in New York City with two guys who ordered the Lumberjack Special (stacks of pancakes wrapped in bacon dunked in butter) at a boutique diner, I ordered oatmeal with strawberries.

Oatmeal with strawberries.

That morning, I took quite a few on the chin about my masculinity. Jibes I could barely hear over the crunch of their crispy bacon and my own sobbing in oatmeal.

But it was actually after that breakfast that something amazing happened.

A full month into being vegan, something felt different. I ate an entire breakfast and felt . . . . great. Full without feeling sick, as if I had just eaten a cloud of happiness. Meanwhile, my mealtime companions were experiencing stomach pains and frequent trips to the bathroom. Was I onto something? Could being vegan really make you feel better about yourself and your choices?

Soon after, I was locked into a pretty good rhythm with my diet—I ate whole grains and mostly plant-based foods with the occasional soy burger or fake chicken patty thrown in. We were also experimenting with other "replacement" foods to satisfy my cravings: pizza by Daiya, spicy tofu wings, sweet potato fries, vegan ice cream, and other delectable vegan treats. Dining remained a challenge, but at this point I was starting to feel the positive effects of eating vegan, and I realized I wasn't going to starve to death.

Then, I had my annual physical.

I had already given blood to the lab so I would be able to discuss my results with my doctor during our appointment. That morning at the doctor's office, I weighed in at 212 pounds (I lost five pounds in the first sixty days) and proceeded to sit across from my doctor to discuss my numbers.

"Hm. Your cholesterol," she said, reviewing the numbers with greater scrutiny, "has dramatically improved: HDL is 53 and LDL is 70. Pretty much cut in half from your last visit." She looked at me as if I'd done something wrong. Checking my blood pressure, she said, "Perfect. 110 over 60. You seem to be doing something right." My pulse rate was 70 and I passed the rest of my exam with flying colors.

"Whatever it is you're doing . . . keep doing it," she remarked.

"I have to," I replied. There was a bet. A bet I refused to lose.

The benefits of being vegan were starting to show in more ways than one, most noticeably when I fastened my belt the following month and had lost four inches in my waist and an additional ten pounds.

And then I watched *Forks Over Knives*. Not since *Weird Science* has a movie had such a long-lasting, profound effect on me. Seeing the evidence and hearing the results plant-based living so prominently portrayed helped to make my short-term bet into a lifelong decision. Plus, meeting T. Colin Campbell in person at a local macro-vegan dinner and hearing his assurances that over time, I will see even more advantages, helped. I was sure that leading a plant-based life was for me.

I started a vegan blog, a vegan business, released my first book based on my blog, *The Skeptical Vegan*, and have worked in marketing for a leading animal rights organization in Washington, DC.

And this all started with a nudge from an eight-year-old.

Kids have much more power than they're given credit for.

Meena's influence changed my life and made me wonder how and when children are told that animals are food. When we explain to children for the first time where meat comes from, their first reaction is often revulsion. They don't want to eat animals. Parents often confront this moral quandary by explaining to children why farm animals have a different role in our lives than other animals.

According to an article published in *Food, Culture and Society*, these family traditions, along with the current pop culture and food advertising influences, "contribute to a food socialization process whereby children learn to conceptually distance the animals they eat from those with whom they have an emotional bond or for whom they feel ethically responsible."

In other words, children learn which animals to love and which to eat, according to accepted social norms. But it doesn't have to be this way. As much as society and outside influences continue to perpetuate this idea, we have a unique opportunity at any stage of life to change perceptions. Perception is reality, after all.

To me, it's as simple as "bite an apple, pet a bunny." Replace the apple with any fruit or vegetable and the bunny with pretty much any animal on the planet. Which will your child choose as food? Which will your child see you picking up and taking a bite out of? Which will they, through your tireless desire to educate, grow emotionally attached to?

I think we all know the answer; it just takes some of us longer to admit it.

Allison Rivers Samson's take on being born compassionate revolves around her vegan daughter, Olivia.

"Our daughter Olivia, who is now eleven, has always been an adept communicator," Allison says. "Before she could speak, we taught her sign language. Early on, she used her signs to convey complex concepts that were well beyond her age.

"When Olivia was about one year old, we visited family in Miami and unwittingly accepted their invitation to Parrot Jungle. As ethical vegans, we choose not to support zoos, circuses, aquatic animal shows, and other events that use animals-in-captivity as entertainment. My husband and I had both grown up in the area and remembered that when we were kids, the birds were free to fly. When we first arrived, that memory was confirmed as we gasped in delight at the sight of the soaring parrots. Phew!

"But that joy was soon dashed. As we rounded a corner, we discovered to our horror that they now had more animals than just birds. And they were kept in cages. I wanted to spare Olivia the sight of a sweet monkey sullenly staring into space as he sat behind bars. But I was too late."

There is never an instance where an animal being kept in a cage, for entertainment or decoration, makes sense. To make a comparison, one only needs to research "human zoos."

Throughout history, and some of it more recent than you'd imagine, humans have been kept in cages and put on display. In 1906, Madison Grant—socialite, eugenicist, amateur anthropologist, and head of the New York Zoological Society—had Congolese pygmy Ota Benga put on display at the Bronx Zoo in New York City alongside apes and other animals.

A human on display at the Bronx Zoo in the twentieth century.

In 1925, a display at Belle Vue Zoo in Manchester, England, entitled "Cannibals" featured Africans who were depicted as savages. Humans on display for the entertainment of other humans. Taking speciesism into account, these same atrocities apply to any sentient being, and, once again, children often pick up on this before adults.

Speciesism [spee-shee-ziz-uh m]
[noun] discrimination in favor of one species, usually the human
species, over another, especially in the exploitation or mistreat-
ment of animals by humans

"Olivia has always had a sixth sense for anyone in distress," Allison continues. "Even at playgroups when another baby was upset, she would sign to me that the other child needed me to nurse him or her since that so often comforted her. This was an early hint at her generous spirit. Even today, she readily shares anything. Even when she has just one or two of something, she will freely give half to someone else.

"This instance at the zoo was no different. As soon as she saw the monkey, Olivia started signing. What she said shocked me. She told me that the monkey was sad and that he didn't want to be there. She wanted us to help him. And how do you think she wanted us to help him? By sharing her mama's milk with him of course!

"Children are born with a compass that points toward compassion. This is why when they discover that the 'food' on their plates was once a living being, many kids denounce eating chickens, pigs, and cows, declaring that they will never do it again. As long as we adults listen and let them lead the way, our children will help us return to our original compassion, too.

"You can support your child's innate kindness while making sure she gets all the nutrients she needs and avoids things that are harmful to her health. Bonus: Following your child's lead will also boost your health and help our planet, too!"

Animals deserve to be free; but what about companion animals? Vegans are sometime criticized for hard-lining the fact that animals should never be caged or kept; meanwhile, they're walking their three dogs on a leash and have left their cat home in a one-bedroom walk-up apartment.

But when talking about lifestyle conflicts and veganism, it seems to me that whether or not vegans should have pets is a question at the heart of what it means to be vegan. If veganism is about treating animals well and fighting against cruelty, then what is wrong with having a pet? There are millions of dogs and cats that need good homes—can you call yourself a true vegan if you *don't* offer to share your home with at least one of these creatures?

And then there's the (bad) argument that farm animals have been domesticated to such a point that we may as well eat them since it's their "purpose" now and they wouldn't exist if humans *didn't* eat them.

Most vegans I know share their lives with pets—many of them, in fact—and their pets do have good lives (evidenced by #dogsofinstragram or #catsofinstagram). The animals and people enjoy each other's company and bring happiness to each other. How can that be a bad thing? This is one issue in the larger vegan worldview that is absolutely indicative of the fact that this lifestyle is not black and white; it's not "all right or all wrong." And it's an ideal that exists in the midst of a nonvegan reality.

Enter Kimchi, our mini poodle mix. We adopted her from the Tompkins County SPCA a few years ago (a month before we all went vegan) after a friend sent us a photo of a very scrappy-looking dog who had been abandoned by her owner. Kimchi needed a home, and we decided the moment we saw her that we wanted to adopt her. As animal rescue advocates, we don't believe in supporting the breeding industry when there are millions of homeless dogs and cats ready to share their love.

As I've mentioned, Kimchi is vegan. Her primary dog food is Natural Balance Vegan formula, and we also prepare our own meals and always set aside some for her. She loves brown rice, quinoa, pasta, kale, broccoli, tofu, and just about anything we give her. Since dogs are omnivores (as opposed to cats, who are true carnivores), she is a very happy and healthy vegan dog. This happiness is shown by her wagging tail and the enthusiasm she greets us with each day.

Unsure about raising your dog vegan? Check out Bramble, a twenty-seven-year-old border collie (189 years old in human years) whose vegan diet of rice, lentils, and organic vegetables earned her consideration by the *Guinness Book of World Records* as the world's oldest living dog back in 2002.

Studies have shown that the ailments associated with meat consumption in humans, such as allergies; cancer; and kidney, heart, and bone problems also affect many nonhumans. Pet food has also been recalled during mad cow disease (or bovine spongiform encephalopathy [BSE]), scares because of the risk that contaminated meat was processed into the food. One deputy commissioner states that cats especially "are susceptible to BSE."

Kimchi thrives on her vegan diet, and we can rest easy knowing that the food scraps dropped by our little ones are just as good for her as they are for them.

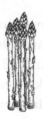

4

RELEARNING THE FOOD PYRAMID: TURN YOUR DINNER TABLE OVER

"The only animals I eat are crackers."
—Anonymous

I've been saying since the introduction that raising vegan kids is not going to be easy. While this statement is completely true, I'd like to take a moment now to say that raising a vegan *from birth* is actually very simple.

Congratulations, you now have a vegan baby! See how easy that was? Now that you've decided to *raise* them vegan, you'll face a myriad of new challenges—challenges that are actually surmountable. Feed them all the vegan foods and teach them to love all animals and not wear or use their byproducts—and, just like that, they're *still* vegan.

However, how would you approach someone trying to convert a kid already on the Standard American Diet (SAD) to a WFPB (whole-food, plant-based) diet?

Dr. Tom Campbell's number one tip is also his second and third tips. "Number one, two, and three is eat a healthy diet *yourself.* Eat what you want them to eat. Both parents need to do this, optimally. That is funda-mental to getting kids to make healthier choices."

It's up to you. So, how *is* your diet? What are you eating that's going to encourage and support your kids' eating habits?

In our household, we make the same meals everyone else in America makes—but we're making the vegan versions of them. Burgers and fries. Pizza and wings. Lasagna and garlic bread. Vegetable stir fry and sushi. These foods, combined with a discipline to make sure we add as many greens onto our plates as possible, are our assurances that our two little ones are eating right. As I said earlier, though, we have it easy since our two toddlers never knew anything else.

"It depends on the kid's age," Dr. Campbell says. "The reality is, unfortunately for the kid, that they are pretty much little prisoners that you love with all your heart. If your young child is otherwise healthy and they don't have a developmental disorder or a disorder related to eating obsessions, you can just limit their choices to healthy options within a well-planned, varied plant-based diet.

"Give them control over which healthy option they want and try to cater to their preferences within healthy options. Get them involved as much as possible in food choice and prep. But the bottom line is that they have to eat what you prepare. And if they don't, they can fast for an evening."

Sound familiar?

"There doesn't need to be a fight or anger or nastiness," Dr. Campbell continues, "but the food served is the food served. There's no backup chicken fingers or French fries that appear if they scream enough. And when they want to eat again, present the food they refused before, and they have to take a few bites. It may seem a bit harsh, but it can work well if it's in a spirit of calm nurturing. Consistency is essential. Never give in to screaming temper tantrums for unhealthy food because that's a clear lesson to your kid that the method works, which they are more than happy to note and use again in the future."

Tough love from Dr. Tom Campbell, and he's right. Your kids may protest for some time, but as you find new foods for them to try and fall in love with, it's the classic situation of "pulling the bandage off fast instead of slow." Start now with better eating, and by the time you're finish reading this book, they'll be vegan.

Campbell also offers, "Sometimes kids aren't going to spend a lot of focus on eating (I'm looking at you, toddlers), and you just need to be sure they get plenty of calories. Don't be shy about offering nuts, nut butters, and avocados. These high-calorie density foods can be your friend.

"Older kids in adolescence, who spend more time independently outside the home, need to have their autonomy respected. But that doesn't mean you have to buy them Twinkies and Oreos (which happen to be vegan) every time you go to the store. It's your money, and you're the parent. You can fill the home environment with only healthy food and get rid of the junk entirely. Make the healthy food convenient, easy, and normative, and then let nature take its course. If they want to continue the junk, they can buy it with their own money. You can discuss and rationalize more with teens, if they are open to it. Discuss why you are eating this way, what you hope the benefits are, and why it's important to you. Sometimes in this age group, environmental or animal welfare arguments make a bigger impact than health arguments. But mostly, it comes down to setting a good example and creating a healthy environment with only healthy options and letting the teen come to you."

So, what should be the first thing eliminated in a soon-to-be-vegan's diet and what are some first steps a parent should consider?

"Honestly, this is a hard question to answer because it depends on the current diet," Campbell says. "If a kid is a junk food eater, mostly vegetarian (loads of sugary, fatty, salty processed foods), and only eating a little yogurt and meat now and then, I'd suggest first putting major emphasis on getting the processed foods out of the diet. The standard American kid diet is so loaded with added sugar, refined flours, and added fats that it's terrible."

This addresses nonvegan junk food, but what are the pitfalls/dangers of falling into a *vegan* junk food trap?

"Processed plant fragments (added sugars and pure fats, as well as refined flours) and the edible products they form are the most nutrient-deficient products you can consume," says Dr. Campbell. "They are fiber-deficient, vitamin-deficient, and mineral-deficient; and they are loaded with empty calories, calories that attack your cardiovascular system and metabolic system, leading to weight gain, diabetes, and rotten teeth. These processed edible products are unnatural technological formulations to create addicts. They are not natural and they will make you sick. Eat what nature (or God, if you prefer) provided. Eat the whole food."

What other tips does Dr. Campbell offer?

"Feeding kids really is about making the same commitment to healthy nutrition and lifestyles in yourself that you want to see in your kids. Start with yourself, and then build an environment that supports your healthy choices. With less pain than you may expect, your kid will follow in your (healthier) footsteps."

Robin Fetter, a mother of three vegan kids, is the CEO, founder, and blogger at *The Real Vegan Housewife* as well as the CEO and founder at Charlottesville Veg Parents Network. A writer at *T.O.F.U. Magazine*, she also has a similar philosophy about her vegan dinner table.

"In my home, there are two options at every meal: 'take it' or 'leave it.' It was the gold standard when I was growing up, and I guess that never left me even when I had kids of my own. Luckily, my kids have no desire to eat animals since they have been vegan all of their lives, but I will admit they probably wish I served them vegan mac 'n' cheese, pizza, and 'chicken' nuggets every day. But even on those days when I serve them something more colorful and whole-foods oriented, they will at least try before they reject it. Anything that is rice and beans, pasta, or on a bed of potatoes is usually a winner for them."

In September 2017, Belgium, a country known mostly for making amazing beer, released a new food pyramid that puts beans, tofu, oils, vegetables, and grains at the top, recommending that these are the foods one should prioritize in their diet. Midway down the food pyramid are eggs, chicken, dairy, and fish; with red meat and butter all the way down at the very bottom. And it gets better—these guidelines put processed meats, like bacon and salami, in a circle that's floating outside the pyramid, along with cakes, cookies, alcohol, and soda. Eat the foods in this bad food satellite "as little as possible," it says. Makes sense. (French fries are also in this "bad food" satellite. I guess they can't get everything right.)

These guidelines, released by the Flemish Institute of Health Life, reflect the 2015 World Health Organization's (WHO) statement that processed meat is now classified as a carcinogen. Combine this with all we know about dairy, and you will get a really clear picture of what we should be putting into our bodies and, more specifically, the bodies of the little ones we care for.

Belgium isn't the first country to recommend dramatic changes to what we've been told in regard to nutrition. The British government recommends that citizens consume less dairy. The Netherlands released a set of dietary guidelines that recommend limits on meat due to sustainability concerns. The Chinese government also released a new set of dietary guidelines that have the potential to see the country's consumption of meat drop by 50 percent. If the average person consumes an average of 70 pounds of meat per year and there are 1,379,000,000 people in China, that means they currently consume 96,530,000,000 pounds of meat. That's 96 billion pounds of meat per year in *one country*.

Thankfully, Belgium's new food guidelines reflect the waves of changes we have seen in the world as more people come to recognize the impact that their food choices have on their own health, the planet, and the animals.

Not surprisingly, the United States government has yet to take such proactive actions in encouraging people to consume less meat and dairy, which is why it's up to you and your offspring to usher in a new generation of vegans. You already know that red meat, and probably eggs, are high in cholesterol and should be avoided to reduce the risk of heart disease—but did you think the same about milk?

Allison River Samson, whose company The Dairy Detox organizes a comprehensive twelve-day program that teaches participants everything they need to know to live and love the dairy-free life, elaborates:

> A cow's milk is designed to fuel massive growth by growing a hundred-pound calf into a thousand-pound cow in the first year of life. The average human growth is from approximately eight pounds to thirty pounds in the same timeframe. Most of

the diseases we have in the developed world are considered diseases of excess, or "over-nutrition."

The NIH (National Institutes of Health) has found that one in three US citizens is overweight or obese. The Centers for Disease Control and Prevention (CDC) states that heart disease is responsible for one in every four US deaths. Eating foods that are high in fat and cholesterol is causing serious consequences to our health, and the common practice of feeding another species's milk to our children is responsible for numerous health afflictions. Eight ounces of 1-percent cow's milk contains 12 milligrams of cholesterol, and more than half of the fat is saturated, while almond milk has zero cholesterol or saturated fat.

But how can we possibly get our calcium without consuming cow's milk? Believe it or not, cow's milk is not the only source of calcium. Have you ever thought about how cows get the calcium that's in their milk? It's in their food—which is 100 percent plants—so just as the cows do, we can get our calcium from plants!

Calcium is found in greens like broccoli, kale, and bok choy; nuts and seeds such as almonds and sesame seeds; kidney beans; and even blackberries. Eating a plant-rich diet and including these foods will help you get the calcium you need, but you can always take a supplement or eat fortified foods to make sure your bases are covered.

Allison also provides insight into lactose intolerance and dairy allergies.

Lactose intolerance is a reaction to milk that is so common that two out of every three adults has it. Even though it's common, not everyone knows what lactose intolerance is. Babies produce an enzyme called lactase that allows them to digest lactose, the sugar in Mom's milk. Once babies wean, most stop producing lactase since they no longer need to digest their mother's milk. Lactose intolerance is the nature-made inability to digest milk beyond the first few years of life.

Parents are increasingly discovering that their children are allergic to milk. Where a milk intolerance is a reaction to the sugar—lactose—a milk allergy is a reaction to the protein—casein. Dairy allergy symptoms can include digestive upsets like colic, spitting up, gas, diarrhea, and even green stools with mucus or blood; skin issues such as mild skin rashes and eczema; and respiratory problems including excessive mucus, runny noses, post-nasal drip, congestion, chronic ear infections, and even more severe problems like asthma and anaphylactic shock.

This is why if a baby is fussy, gassy, or has skin or digestive issues, cow's milk and other dairy products are the first foods a doctor will recommend removing from a nursing mother's diet since anything she eats can transfer into her milk and directly to her baby. It's easy to see that the only way dairy lives up to its marketing campaign title, "nature's perfect food," is if you're a baby cow.

Kristina Parker is a vegan mom raising her two-year old son, Colin, with her husband in Portland, Oregon. As a new vegan, she had a huge learning curve, but she feels very supported by her in-law family and her local community. Portland is a vegan's paradise.

When I visited Portland for a few days on business, I was amazed at the vast number of vegan options, from food trucks (check out DC Veg and Homegrown Smoker) to bars (visit The Sweet Hereafter and Blackwater). Portland is also where I consumed my first vegan donut (Voodoo Doughnut), which was bigger than my head. When you're vegan *for the animals*, you can eat whatever you want—as long as you're not allergic to any of the ingredients.

Since deciding to become vegan in the spring of 2017, Kristina's husband, sister, in-laws, and even her nanny all expressed interest and have decided to start this lifestyle with her. She feels very blessed that her journey to plant-based living has started early on in her son's life at just two years of age. The thing is, baby Colin has food allergies to dairy, eggs, and cashews, which include two of the three main food groups vegans avoid in the first place.

"At two months old, Colin started getting severe reactions, including full body rashes, reflux, and blood in his GI tract," Kristina says. "I was breastfeeding at the time and embarked on an elimination diet from the top eight allergens. We discovered that dairy was a major aggravator, and I continued a dairy-free diet. At around four months old, I also eliminated eggs after noticing patterns of previous symptoms returning. Colin's health status started to slowly improve. This experience primed me to look for future allergy reactions to foods.

"As Colin got older and we introduced solid foods, he had a severe reaction to scrambled eggs at a restaurant. This prompted an urgent visit to the pediatrician and a prescription for EpiPen Jr®. We discovered the cashew allergy after becoming vegan and trying a cashew-based Alfredo sauce for pasta. Colin broke out with blisters on his face immediately. He has now been tested with an Ig-E blood test to help monitor his allergy status."

In spite of all of this, Kristina is still committed to a vegan household.

"The allergy reactions we've experienced have changed my perspective of food. We found so many replacements for our diet and are content living without them. This led me to challenge why we consume any animal products at all and to dive deeper into our awareness of what we put into our bodies for food. The decision to become vegan is such a good fit for our family values, including: teaching the importance of compassion and empathy for all living beings; providing a plant-based nutrition foundation for my son and his future; and raising a conscious son that is aware of global environmental, ethical, and health impacts of his food choices.

"I love the deeper connection I have with animals now, and the opportunity to share that with Colin, especially at animal sanctuaries."

The strategy for approaching both Colin's allergies as well as his vegan diet with pediatricians and family members also showed Kristina's unwavering commitment to stay vegan.

"When discussing allergens with Colin's pediatrician, we are given a lot of freedom to direct what we want to do (in terms of re-introducing allergens to his diet). I used to experience anxiety about starting a baked milk or baked egg challenge. I am glad to share our story of becoming plant-based with the medical community now and focusing on preventative health. This shift has given me the perspective that nutrition is our first medicine.

"With family and friends, we can confidently share our story of transitioning to veganism as a family. I share that our initial challenge was finding a diet that eliminated eggs and dairy for Colin, and that this led us to eliminate animal products completely. In addition, we have found a lifestyle that fits our values."

I'd love to check in on Kristina's family in another five years to see how it's going and how much Colin is thriving. Her thoughtful and devoted approach to going vegan is precisely the kind of story I can relate to, and I would love to continue sharing with others.

Allergies are one thing we all learn to avoid or work around, but what about general food safety unrelated to hypersensitivity?

While doing research for this book, I stumbled on an ad for "Pennsalt Chemicals" from 1947, and I honestly thought it was a parody. The ad featured a retro illustration of a housewife, happy farm animals, colorful food, and a dog—all dancing and singing the praises of *Dichlorodiphenyltrichloroethane* (DDT). In this fun-filled, full-page, full-color ad, DDT is depicted as the answer to all the world's problems.

DDT is now illegal. In fact, the ban on DDT in the United States is partly responsible for the comeback of the American bald eagle from the endangered species list.

Back in the day, DDT was used for everything, from agricultural sprays to household pesticides. The US was just coming off a high of its own, having defeated (with the Allies) the Axis powers in World War II just a couple of years earlier. It was time for this country to innovate and support the blossoming baby boom. What better way to do that than to take hazardous materials and introduce them into our daily lives? America was aglow with opportunity, and DDT was (as the ad claims):

- Good for fruits: Making them bigger and free from worms! Who doesn't want a bigger apple?

- Good for steers: They'll grow bigger cows, too, because of DDT. Bigger, like in Texas.
- Good for homes: That's right, sprinkle some DDT in your kid's nursery to chase away those pests!
- Good for dairies: Now that we're about to go big with this milk thing, gotta figure out how to make more milk! DDT!
- Good for row crops: We're pushing out the taters in numbers never seen before!
- Good for industry: Pennsalt Products is going to make industry in America strong!

Does all of this sound somewhat familiar? Monsanto, one of the companies that originally manufactured DDT, is the target of much debate and protest today for similar actions. This ad for DDT is almost seventy years old. Like Pennsalt, Monsanto is placing its genetically modified products on store shelves before researchers have a total understanding of their scientific impact. The cycle continues.

Since then, DDT has been shown to damage the nervous, immune, endocrine, and neurological systems, not to mention its devastating influence on the natural environment. DDT was being introduced into our foods without our approval as far back as the 1940s. So, to those of you standing up against Monsanto and thinking that GMOs, food science, and tampering with what you eat is a new thing—think again. It's as old as your mother.

Moving along alphabetically and sticking with the acronym theme, let's go from DDT to GMO. It seems like everyone, and vegans are much to blame, is talking about the dangers of genetically modified organisms (GMOs) these days. We want to know what's in our food. But what are GMOs exactly, and do they impact the vegan diet? What is the future of safe food?

GMOs are the result of a laboratory process that inserts genes from one species into the genes of another to obtain a desired trait or characteristic; for example, fast-growing seafood like salmon. However, GMOs are actually as prevalent in a vegan diet. In fact, among the top ten GMO foods to avoid, all but one (dairy) are vegan. Corn tops the list, followed by soy and sugar.

So, what can you do if you're trying to avoid genetically-modified foods? *Always* try to buy organic (although even doing that is no guarantee), know the source of your foods, and look for the "Non-GMO Verified" label. As you continue to load up on fruits and veggies, keep in mind that *most* fresh produce is naturally non-GMO, but zucchini, yellow summer squash, edamame, sweet corn, and papaya from Hawaii or China are considered high risk and are best avoided. Only buy those high-risk fruits and vegetables if they are labeled "organic" or "non-GMO."

Since GMOs currently require no labeling, most companies won't tell us what foods do have GMOs. So when these seals are used, you can be sure that those foods are GMO-free.

However, notice that I didn't write "safe from GMOs," since GMOs haven't actually been deemed unsafe. In fact, two friends of mine, who are both Cornell biologists, believe in GMOs and feel that they are the answer to world hunger. They also tell me that *everything* we eat has been GMOed at some point in time, so they're essentially unavoidable anyway.

Does all this GMO talk stress you out? Do you want to feed your little one the best food possible? Take a deep breath, and just start with baby steps. Don't feel overwhelmed—just do the best you can and start eliminating GMOs however you can for just a couple of weeks and pay close attention to your health, weight, energy, and mood. Also take note of your kid's health and attention spans. See what positive changes are taking effect, if you notice any, by being on a non-GMO diet, and go from there.

Nothing tastes as good as healthy feels.

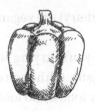

5

VEGANIZING YOUR HOLIDAYS: SANTA AIN'T VEGAN, BUNNIES DON'T LAY EGGS, AND THE HALLOWEEN SWITCH WITCH

"No one has ever become poor by giving."
—*Anonymous*

Ah, Christmas! The beloved holiday where you stand, bleary-eyed, for hours in the toy section at Target at 11:00 p.m., randomly grabbing anything that costs less than ten dollars, the last roll of the Paw Patrol wrapping paper, scattered ribbons and bows, and a six-pack of tape. All in a blur of exhaustion on Christmas Eve.

Santa Claus ain't gonna buy those toys for you. Besides, he wouldn't make a very good personal shopper anyway since Santa ain't vegan.

Let's start with his clothes. I'm pretty sure his red suit is made of 100 percent wool, his belt is made from leather, and his boxers are made from silk. Wool, leather, and silk are all not vegan items. Add to this the fact that Santa Claus has a known cookie and milk addiction, and we can all assume that those *aren't* vegan cookies or plant-based milks.

And, of course, Santa Claus regularly reins rambunctious reindeer to what must be a one-ton sled and forces them to fly his fat ass around the world delivering gifts—all in one night.

Someone should turn him over to the Humane Society of the United States (HSUS). He's obviously in direct contravention of numerous animal rights mandates. Let's not even talk about those poor elves barely making a living wage and working countless overtime hours.

Christmas is demanding, as is Thanksgiving, Hanukkah, and Independence Day (barbecues). All holidays are challenging holidays for vegan families for different reasons. Most focus attention on a "roast" of some sort or another animal-centric centerpiece. Luckily, most of these sides circulating around it are already vegan, and roasts can be made with plant-based ingredients or you can serve a store-bought version.

Thanksgiving has always been my favorite holiday. Baste all morning. Cook all day. Eat for thirty minutes. Lounge. After we went vegan, we had a new challenge: how to deal with Thanksgiving when certain family members insist on eating meat. Try as we might, we invited my mom to our house for a vegan Thanksgiving, but she insisted on bringing meat. We were then invited to her house, where she insisted on eating meat. Needless to say, we had to rethink our usual traditions and learn to celebrate a compassionate holiday with newfound vegan friends.

These days, Thanksgiving is still my favorite holiday, with all the basting, cooking, eating, and lounging intact. Each year we host, or co-host, a vegan Thanksgiving (known in the vegan circles as ThanksLiving), inviting many other families, each of whom bring their own vegan kids.

As soon as the foil is taken off the food, the Hungry Youngsters (band name) swoop in like voracious vultures and devour everything. Usually, I can't grab my camera fast enough to get photographic proof that the meal actually existed. We stand back and watch the food evaporate and give thanks that we are able to eat well for the holidays and celebrate with good friends.

Our usual holiday fare looks a lot like this—and trust me, no one ever leaves hungry or ever misses meat:

Celebration Roast: Stuffed with cornbread stuffing. The perfect centerpiece to the table. Ours is homemade (comprised mostly of tofu) and happens to be the exact size and shape of our spaghetti strainer.

Mashed potatoes: Clearly the most popular dish, in spite of the fact that it broke the "no nightshades" rule. Nightshades are foods like peppers and potatoes that some people have an adverse reaction to. With this said, mashed potatoes are very easily veganized since there are vegan butters and alt-milks to smooth out the taters. What kid doesn't love mashed potatoes?

Chipotle scalloped sweet potatoes: Sweet and hot and orange. What more would you want in a food? You can also turn it down a notch and leave out the chipotle.

Cranberries: Had to have them. Their sweet and tart flavor balances so well against the savory foods. When I was a kid, this dish was always shaped like a can for some reason.

Penne Alfredo: My old standby. Creamy and full of basil. I think I need to start calling this "pesto Alfredo." It's another one of those "cheesy" dishes our kids love.

Roasted Brussels sprouts: I love Brussels sprouts. They are like tiny cabbages (which is actually what they are). Whenever I eat them, I feel like a giant. So will your kids.

Noodle Kugel: The perfect addition to the Thanksgiving/Hanukkah mashup. We'll have this the next time these two holidays coincide on the same date, in another twenty thousand years.

Kale salad (of course): Always a great dish to bring to any vegan dinner. Vegans love kale. All hail kale.

Gravy: 'nuff said. I always make four quarts (think of this as vegan cream of mushroom soup, since that's essentially what it is). Making vegan gravy made me realize two things: 1) Non-animal gravy doesn't harden into a disgusting lump of fat the day after. It stays smooth and edible, as is. 2) Leftover gravy blended with rice makes the most amazing Thanksgiving-themed risotto. Add that to your leftover repertoire.

Four different pies and ice "cream" for dessert: Apple and butternut squash pies and two flavors of ice cream (one ice cream features my favorite Gimme! Coffee). Obviously, the toughest part about having delicious desserts at any gathering is hiding them until the kids have eaten dinner.

There is truly a reason to celebrate when you know you are eating with a group of twenty or more who all share the same passion for compassion.

One animal rights activist and friend of mine whom I've never spent Thanksgiving with, but would love to, is Rae Sikora.

Rae has been a spokesperson for animals, the environment, and human rights for over thirty years. Her programs have changed people's ideas of what is possible to create in our lives and in the world. Rae has worked internationally with participants ranging from teachers, students, and prisoners to businesses and activists.

I'm also one of a growing number of compassionate people who can call Rae a friend. I first met her at Summerfest, the annual four-day vegan meetup in Johnstown, Pennsylvania, which takes place around July 4. It brings together all the thought leaders in vegan nutrition as well as animal rights activists, and it is the one event I would most encourage you to attend—with your kids. Summerfest is an experience the entire family would love and learn from; plus the vegan food is amazing.

Rae is a ray of sunshine, one of the warmer and more wonderful vegans I've ever known. When I told Rae I was working on this book, I asked her to add her own comments to the chapter about Thanksgiving, since I knew she would be able to articulate how I feel about this annual holiday and its impact on the animals. She says:

Thanksgiving. The holiday where many progressive and socially conscious types have already ordered their "organic" or "pasture-raised" turkeys, allowing them to eat the traditional meal without the guilt of supporting factory farming and chemical-laden agriculture. However, most well-intentioned people won't look any further to discover the truth behind their meal.

Organic standards do not include regulations about the treatment of the animals. Rae continues:

A friend and I visited a local organic farm with a good reputation for environmental and humane standards. The farm's reputation seemingly held true. Their one thousand birds are raised in large outdoor hoop-houses with green pasture surrounding. Their feed is organically grown on the farm and hangs from feeders accessible to any of the birds who are able to walk to them. They even slaughter the birds right on the farm, avoiding transport to a large slaughterhouse facility.

Yet even under "better than average" conditions, the turkeys suffer. Most people ordering organic birds assume they are not genetically bred for weight gain. Organic and non-organic turkeys are bred to be slaughter-ready at eighteen weeks. They are so obese that their legs cannot handle the weight of their bodies. In fact, many birds are completely lame by two months.

Some of the turkeys we saw were stuck in the straw, unable to get up, and struggling to make it to food and water while healthier birds pecked at them. Others, already dead, were being removed.

Our tour guide, the farm manager of eleven years, was kind and open with us. He told us he was proud of the facility and happy to show us around. In the slaughter building, we were introduced to a worker he nicknamed "the killer." The manager chuckled and said they actually, "refer to him as the 'harvester.'" I asked the young harvester if his job was difficult. Thoughtfully, he replied, "It was hard at first, but it gets easier."

They then showed us the procedure. The birds are "gently" pushed into wall-mounted funnels head first and upside down. With their heads hanging below an opening at the base of the funnel, the "harvester" slices the major arteries on the bird's neck. A bucket catches the blood below. In the words of the harvester, "I slice with a clean hundred-dollar surgical knife. I am careful not to cut the airway. We need them alive, breathing, and bleeding to drain all the blood out or it gets too messy in the next step. It is very fast. It only takes two minutes. They are breathing the whole time and their legs are kicking."

I stood there struck by his words "only two minutes." I recently led a workshop where I wanted people to guess how long a minute is. Everyone closed their eyes. I told the participants to open their eyes and raise their hands when they thought a minute was up. I timed them. Almost everyone had their eyes open and hands raised in about thirty seconds. A minute is a long time. Two minutes of hanging upside down with your major arteries sliced open and bleeding is a really long time.

After touring the entire facility, from pasture to the freezer filled with hundreds of tidy, packaged birds, we walked slowly back to my car feeling distressed by our experience. I have met some "used-to-be vegetarians" who have turned to a meat diet again because of the availability of animal products labeled "humane." Everyone who chooses to eat animal products labeled "humane," "cage-free," "organic," or "free-range" should visit the facility providing their meat, dairy, or eggs. Anyone wanting to live compassionately would not support these industries. They would hopefully realize that these labels give people permission to turn their backs on the violent reality of eating these foods. The creation of all animal products involves exploitation for profit including confinement, social deprivation, mutilation, reproductive manipulation, and premature death.

Make your next Thanksgiving a ThanksLiving by modifying tradition to include nonviolence toward all beings and caring for the earth and your own health.

I was reading bedtime stories to our little vegan boy when I came across the veganesque poem "Point of View" in the collection *Where the Sidewalk Ends* by Shel Silverstein. I've probably read this book a hundred times over the years, but this time the poem, which portrays the point of view of the "dinner" served at the table, had so much more meaning to me. For example, to a turkey, Thanksgiving is "sad and thankless." It's perfect for the holiday season and something you'll want to share with your kids.

Shel would have made a great vegan.

Traditional family holidays can be challenging to new vegans, and there's probably not one more challenging than the holiday that literally involves kids dressed in disguise and begging total strangers for candy. Halloween—insert "doom doom *doom*" music.

If possible, stay home on Halloween. When that's not an option, which is probably always, here are some tips and tricks tried and true from vegan parents around the globe.

How do vegan parents deal with trick or treating? What tricks can they use to keep the treats vegan while still keeping the holiday fun for the kids?

Robyn Moore, mother to a four-year-old boy, says that it's cute seeing him come into his own about what he calls being a "bēgan." She also has a seven-year-old girl who asked if water was vegan when she first started exploring it.

Kids say the darndest things, and vegan kids say even cuter, darnder things. Paisley, our three-year-old going on thirteen-year-old, calls tofu "toe food." Luckily, she still loves eating it.

Robyn has a master's degree in education and a certificate in plant-based nutrition from Cornell University, and she is currently pursuing a certificate in humane education. She is working with the Institute for Humane Education to open the Solutionary School New York City. She is the creator of the website and blog *RaisingVegKids*, the organizer of NYC Vegetarian & Vegan Families Meetup, and a book reviewer for *Vegbooks*. Robyn has worked hard at creating her own vegan community, and she is surrounded by numerous vegan parents who have risen to their own challenges.

Such as how to deal with the mother of all vegan challenges, Halloween.

"There are a few easy options that vegan parents have developed when it comes to Halloween," Robyn says. "The reality is that when kids trick or treat, nonvegan candy will end up in their bags. I've heard the argument that it's only one day, and you should just let your kids eat the nonvegan candy; but I disagree with that. First of all, it's not just one day; kids end up eating their candy for weeks. But more important, it sends the wrong message that it's okay to eat nonvegan food/candy if it's part of a celebration or other event."

And I agree. It's a very slippery slope once you start allowing your kids to consume nonvegan foods, especially chocolate and candy. So, what do you do with all that nonvegan candy that's inevitably going to end up in your kids' pumpkin bucket?

"You have two choices; you can either donate the candy to homeless shelters, nursing homes, and employees at animal shelters, or bring it to work to give to colleagues," Robyn recommends. "Dentist offices are even participating in a program that buys your leftover Halloween candy and sends it to the troops overseas. Personally, in our house, we just throw out all the nonvegan candy because it's sugary, nutrient-deficient junk anyway and isn't good for anybody.

"After you've separated out all the nonvegan candy, if there's not much vegan candy left, you might consider adding in some more that you've bought ahead of time for exactly this situation! Have some of your kids' favorite ones, like Skittles, Dum-Dums, Twizzlers, Smarties, Swedish Fish, Jolly Ranchers, and Dots, and maybe even surprise them with an extra special treat like a vegan peep from one of the online vegan companies."

(By the way, if you want to support a family-owned candy company where one of the owners is both a woman and an ethical vegan, buy Smarties. Liz Dee and her sisters are co-presidents of this seventy-year-old New Jersey–based candy company *and* she's also a powerful voice in the vegan community.)

"I've even made vegan candy corn—from a recipe online—that tasted just like the original," Robyn continues. "For many kids, Halloween is mostly about dressing up and having fun, so don't deprive them of this experience because of the few nonvegan candies that might end up in their bag. Remember that your kids have to go to school the next day and hear about all of the candy the other kids got, and you want your kid to be able to participate in that conversation and excitedly share what they received. This helps further the idea that veganism isn't a sacrifice and kids don't have to miss out on any fun. Think about it, if nonvegan classmates heard that they couldn't trick or treat on Halloween, do you think they'd want to be vegan?

"Another option of getting rid of the nonvegan candy your kid has collected is the Switch Witch. It's a fun new idea that's catching on with families everywhere—not only by vegans, but also conscious parents looking to limit their kids' consumption of sugary junk. At night, kids leave the nonvegan candy in a bag by their bedroom door (or front door), and the Switch Witch flies in and takes it. In its place, she leaves a gift. There's even a cute book *Switchcrafted: The Story of The Switch Witches of Halloween Book* to go along with this—we did it when my daughter was very young. I'd recommend it for kids under five. It's a great solution that allows kids to participate in the quintessential Halloween experience, while still sticking to their vegan values."

Here's a film idea: *Halloween: Attack of the Vegans!*

EXT. MAIN STREET USA, NIGHT

Young VEGAN KIDS celebrating Halloween night. VEGAN KIDS ring the doorbell of a home with spider webs, pumpkins, and skeletons. They wait. The door opens as the HOMEOWNER [WOMAN, MID-FIFTIES] opens the creaky door.

KIDS: Trick or treat!

HOMEOWNER: Aw. You two look cute in your, um, what is that? A Daiya cheese bag costume? And, what have we here? Oh, you're an avocado. How adorable.

[HOMEOWNER drops candy into two outstretched hemp bags]

KID 1: Is this candy vegan?

HOMEOWNER: Yes! As a matter of . . .

KID 2: Is it organic?

HOMEOWNER: Why, yes!

KID 1: Is it fair trade?

HOMEOWNER: Uh, yeah?

KID 2: But . . . is the wrapper compostable?

HOMEOWNER: I give up.

HOMEOWNER slams door. And . . . scene.

In our home, after hitting up all the houses we can before 7:00 p.m., we do a variation of the Switch Witch that our kids love. We dump out all their bounty on the living room floor and sort the candy into two piles: "vegan" and "not vegan." This becomes an incredible teaching moment, too. The vegan pile is put back into their pumpkin bucket and the non-vegan candy is given to the Switch Witch.

One of us leaves the room with the nonvegan candy and, presto, we reappear minutes later with all *new* vegan candy. Our kids are actually more excited about how this magic happens than having any feelings of missing out or not getting the original candy.

We then give the nonvegan candy to teachers, older kids who are not vegan, or friends who don't have kids. Nothing really goes to waste, and by the end of the night, our kids have the same amount of candy—and we know it's all vegan.

"If you want to skip trick-or-treating altogether, you could host a fun Halloween party, or you could have your kids decorate the house and hand out candy," Robyn adds. "Besides the nonvegan candy, the rest of Halloween is 100 percent vegan fun and really all about dressing up in cool costumes, spooky decorations, and creepy movies; so focus on that."

Kids come in all size, shapes, and colors, and each one has their own unique dietary restriction (note: "picky eater" is not a dietary restriction).

"My six-year-old daughter went trick-or-treating with four friends last year," Robyn says. "My daughter is vegan. One friend was nut-free and another was gluten-free. They all knew exactly what candies they could and couldn't eat. This shows that food becomes part of kids' lives. They don't have to keep reinventing the wheel; they pretty much already know what they can eat. So, after every apartment (we live in New York City), they traded candies with each other. For apartments that just left bowls out, they reached in and grabbed exactly what they could eat. Sometimes there was nothing safe for them in the bowl and it was no biggie; they just turned around and went to the next door. Easy, peasy. But they giggled and ran and had so much fun the whole night, and they all managed to bring home full bags."

Fast forward four months, and you're suddenly face-to-whisker with a basket-leaving rabbit that, for some reason, lays chocolate eggs.

If you celebrate Easter, there are at least three traditions that come to mind that are very nonvegan: egg coloring, egg hunts, and Easter baskets. None of these have anything to do with Jesus, which has always seemed very strange to me.

Little known fact: former California governor and terminal Terminator, Arnold Schwarzenegger, loves Easter. He's been known to say, "Have to love Easter, baby." (I promise, this is the last time I'll use a joke like this for the rest of this book. Maybe.)

When I was a kid, Easter baskets had always been a combination of an oversized hollow chocolate bunny, small bags of jelly beans and candy, a Mad magazine, and a kite—all resting on some fake grass. Luckily, all of these items are available in their vegan versions.

Egg coloring is probably the most challenging of these traditions to veganize, but, as with anything else you want to veganize, it's not impossible. You can always make edible decorative "eggs" by making a batch of vegan sugar cookie dough (there are many recipes on the Internet), roll it out, and cut out egg shapes using an oval cookie cutter. You can then decorate the baked, cooled, egg-shaped cookies with your favorite colored vegan icings and frostings or vegan jimmies.

You can also find unfinished wooden eggs in a variety of sizes at most craft stores. Paint them as you would regular eggs using acrylic paints, which are mostly vegan. If you want to make it fancy, use two differently colored wood stains. There are wood stains available that are nontoxic, effective, beautiful, and durable, with low or no volatile organic compounds (VOC). Some are even food-grade for toys, counter-tops, salad bowls, and kids' furniture.

Then, there are ceramic eggs. These were actually invented for kids with egg allergies, and your vegan kid may just as well pretend they have an egg allergy anyway (it makes ordering food and dealing with school lunches that much easier). You can color them with the same vinegar/color combination you'd use on chicken eggs. And since they're not real chicken eggs, you can invite a chicken over to help.

Hosting a vegan egg hunt is easy and much more fun for the littles than a traditional egg hunt. Go to your local dollar store and load up on those hollow colorful plastic eggs that can open up, along with a dozen or so tiny toys. Little plastic cars, dolls, stickers, etc. Put the goodies inside the eggs and hide them in the yard (if it's warm enough) or in the living room (if it's too cold). This activity can last as long as the level of creative hiding places you've found allows.

(Tell them there are thirteen eggs to find, but only hide twelve.)

Allison River Samson says, "Easter can be a time to honor new beginnings and rebirth in our own lives and in nature all around us. What better way to celebrate life than by holding Easter events that are kind to everyone by being animal-friendly?

"There are plenty of cruelty-free alternatives to the typical Easter activity of dying chickens' eggs. This tradition can be upgraded to decorating wooden eggs that can become family keepsakes or having a vegan Easter egg hunt with plastic eggs filled with treats/stickers.

"Sharing a vegan brunch with family and friends will add a delicious finish to your Easter celebration."

If you celebrate Purim, the Jewish tradition that goes by the Yiddish name *shalach manos*, you are probably accustomed to people giving their friends and neighbors candy and other sweet foodstuffs. Just let your friends and neighbors know in advance that you're vegan and see if they can accommodate. If it seems like a hassle to them, skip their house or bring vegan candy ahead of time to share.

On Chanukah, it is traditional to give children Chanukah *gelt*, which is Yiddish for *money* and has been replaced in recent years with gold chocolate coins. You can find vegan versions of these online (made from dark chocolate), which are gluten-free and with no added sugar.

There are really no holiday traditions your vegan kids will miss out on by being vegan. In fact, they'll learn to appreciate the little things even more. Like when Cooper, our five-year-old who talks nonstop, gave random thanks for our washer and dryer.

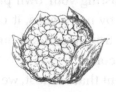

6

BIRTHDAY PARTY PLANNING: BYOC (BRING YOUR OWN CUPCAKES)

"The love for all living creatures is the most noble attribute of man."
—*Charles Darwin*

Vegan holidays are challenging enough—and vegan birthday parties are no piece of cake.

Inevitably, you're most likely going to come across at least two nonvegan food items at nearly every kid's birthday party: cake and pizza. Two items that can be dealt with with two words: *come prepared.*

Just like you'd bring the host of an adult party a bottle of wine or an appetizer to share, you'll also want to bring your own vegan cake (or cupcakes) and vegan pizza to a toddler's birthday party. Parties are chaotic enough without having to forage for food for your kids or to keep their little fingers out of the frosting, all while everyone else is partying and not thinking twice about what they're eating.

Just be prepared and plan on it. Even if you have a hunch that the hosts are going to hook you up, *come prepared.* Trust me, better safe than starving.

Of course, if you're hosting your own party, it's easy. But if you're attending a party hosted by nonvegans, it can be a challenge. But it's nothing some sage advice from vegan-kid-birthday-party-expert Robyn Moore can't help you overcome.

"First, any party or event that we host, we keep it 100 percent vegan," says Robyn, who now boasts as many as eleven vegan birthday parties between her two children, on top of birthday parties for other family members and friends. "It's our party, so it should reflect our values. We want our nonvegan guests to have fun and enjoy the food, so we go the extra mile by providing food that we think will be a hit.

"We tend to rely on food that we've already tested and love, rather than experimenting and trying out new recipes with rare ingredients—we save that for our vegan friends. We serve things that they're already familiar with (so they don't feel like they've taken a rocket ship to another planet), such as chips, crackers, veggies and hummus dip, fruit, pastas, sorbet, etc. Then we choose foods from some of our favorite vegan brands and serve those. If it's a barbeque, of course we'll have veggie dogs and burgers, and we'll make sure to have the best vegan cheese for them to try."

With companies like Beyond Meat, Tofurky, Daiya, and Gardein, you can easily serve burgers, fries, pizza, macaroni and cheese, and chicken nuggets to a hungry mob of kids. These vegan versions of the classics taste exactly like their nonvegan counterparts, and kids gobble them up without batting an eye. Of course, you'll also want to provide ketchup, vegan ranch dressing, and vegan bleu cheese dressing just to keep the party extra clean and tidy.

"As far as going to someone else's party or event that is nonvegan, we haven't really had many issues at all," Moore says. "Ninety percent of the time, the host knows we are vegan and will have something available for us to eat. I usually email ahead of time, too, just to see what they're serving—and then I can bring the same, just in a vegan version."

We've had similar luck with birthday parties our kids have been invited to. I feel that the thoughtful parent appreciates the reminder that we're coming with not one, but two, little vegan party animals.

In some cases, the hosts have gone so far as to make the whole party vegan, knowing that their own kids will still have fun and that putting out vegan treats means they'll also cover most major allergies at the same time (i.e., no eggs or dairy).

If a dozen kids are jumping around at a party and are suddenly offered cake, pizza, and ice cream, there is a 99.9 percent chance they're not going to notice it's vegan.

"I used to try and 'match' the food, but I found out they don't care," says Robyn. "So I just ask them what they want, and they tell me. It's usually pizza, and I bring that. If the other kids at the party are eating chicken sliders, they still want the pizza. The bottom line is we never show up hungry without food of our own. That's just not fair to our kids. We always come prepared with some snacks, at least.

"I think so many vegan parents have this fear—and even I did in the beginning—that their kids will feel left out at parties. In all honesty, this has never been the case. Most of the time, the kids are running around playing, and food is an afterthought. Kids don't really care about food that much; it's the parents who do. They sit and have a few bites of pizza and cake, and then they run off. Most don't even notice what everyone else is eating. Nowadays, so many kids have allergies, so my kids are rarely the only ones eating something different."

Since our littlest little is both vegan *and* gluten-free with her diet, we usually come with a vegan gluten-free pizza. Nine times out of ten another parent will sniff out what we've brought and ask if their child can have some—since they didn't *come prepared.*

"My kids have always been happy to have their food, and especially their cupcake, which they've usually either picked out ahead of time or helped me make. It makes them extra proud to eat it," Robyn says. "When they have school parties, I try to pack a beautiful, big cupcake, and my kids come home saying the other kids wanted theirs! As parents choosing this lifestyle for our kids, it's our responsibility to make sure we are prepared."

What about letting your kids have some leeway when it comes to special events? Can they eat just a single nonvegan cupcake or one slice of pizza?

"No! I think allowing kids to have nonvegan foods once in a while sends the wrong message," Robyn stresses. "It's like dropping your morals at the door and picking them back up after the party. It doesn't make sense. Especially at parties or special events, which is worse because it sets the issue up as 'because we're at this special celebration, you get to do something special like have a nonvegan treat.' It sends a mixed message—a nonvegan treat becomes a positive reward. It downplays the seriousness and importance of why our family is choosing this lifestyle.

"We teach our kids to make decisions based on compassion, not convenience. That said, this is not to be confused with striving for perfection. If my kids were to mistakenly eat something nonvegan, it's not the end of the world. However, we would never knowingly do it."

A kid's birthday party takes some planning, so the first thing you need to do is decide if it's worth the effort. Don't go all out for a one- or even a two-year-old; they have no idea what's going on. A three-year-old will probably start to get the gist, and as for all ages above—yeah, you're going to have to do something special and throw a party.

The second thing you need to figure out is the details. As with anything in life, keeping it as simple as possible will help with your anxiety level. Assuming your child's party is happening at your home, you will be in charge of everything. This means it'll be easy making sure everything is vegan. Grab some family members and friends to help so you can delegate tasks and not run yourself ragged.

It's important to know how many people will attend, so you can plan on the right amount of food—establish an online evite so attendees can send an RSVP via email. If it's a dish-to-pass, link it to a Google sheet for everyone to fill out the foods they plan to bring. If you want to keep the party totally vegan, let your guests know in advance that they need to bring plant-based foods. Make it easier for them by suggesting specific dishes or beverages. If they're truly terrified of trying to make something vegan, list other items they can contribute, such as juice boxes, ice, decorations, or balloons.

Or wine. Let's be honest, you may need it.

Though you and your household are now vegan, taking into account other guests' dietary restrictions, food allergies, and preferences is still very important and guests might have life-threatening nut allergies. So, it's a good idea to label your food.

Something to keep in mind when decorating: balloons are made out of rubber, and rubber is petroleum-based, and petroleum is a by-product of extinct dinosaurs, and dinosaurs were animals. So, balloons aren't vegan.

This is what's known as vegan humor.

All that said, choose eco-friendly decorations, plates, and serving utensils that won't outlive your own time on the planet. There are some great corn-based and biodegradable disposables on the market, and while they may not feature an image of Lightning McQueen, they're better for the planet.

Create a fun playlist with upbeat music, maybe a few songs by vegan musicians (Moby, Bryan Adams, or Carrie Underwood) or songs that are about animals (in a good way, not the "Old McDonald" way). Decorations can play off the recycled/vegan/caring-for-the-Earth theme while adding a festive and fun flare to the event. The excellent website EcoPartyTime.com sells some pretty cool "earthy" party supplies.

Now, on to the cake.

A vegan birthday cake is one of the most important parts of any birthday party. It really becomes the center of attention (as far as I'm concerned, anything covered in frosting or gravy usually becomes the center of attention). Everyone gathers around, sings "Happy Birthday," and watches as the birthday boy or girl makes a wish and blows out the candles—and then smashes their filthy hands into the icing.

You basically have two options for birthday cakes: order a vegan cake from a local bakery or co-op, or make your own. Surprisingly, making your own is very simple since the replacement ingredients (applesauce, almond milk, and vegan butter) are already in your fridge. Most all cake mixes on the market are already vegan, so follow the same directions for baking, but replace the ingredients (eggs, milk, and butter) with their vegan counterparts above—and you've just made a cake.

Color your cake frosting with Watkins food coloring, which is made colorful by plants.

Another option is a vegan cheesecake from Daiya. These taste so much like dairy cheesecakes that both kids and parents alike ask for seconds; and they come in a variety of flavors. You may want to buy two as they're on the small side.

I've eaten a whole cheesecake by myself; I thought it was a single serving package.

Of course, you also have to establish a party theme. While you may be tempted to pick out Elmo or *Frozen*, it could be more fun (and accidentally educational) to choose a theme that relates to animals or veganism. Even something as simple as the films *Finding Nemo* or *Bambi* have a vegan message. Other ideas could be wild animals, animals on the brink of extinction, or farm animals who are free to roam around.

The party theme doesn't have to be printed on new or made-to-order cups, plates, hats, and favor bags. Sometimes just a suggestion of the theme is enough, using items you already own or ones you can borrow from a friend—for example, stuffed animals that are placed around the venue or eco craft items that can make themed decorations. Use colors—blue and orange for Nemo, tan and green for Dora the Explorer, etc.—to help with the thematic suggestion, instead of finding items that use the specific face of a cartoon character. Avoid using materials that are bad for the environment—balloons, plastic cups, disposable flatware, plastic cutouts, etc. If you're left with no choice, be sure to save the decorations so they can be reused by other parents.

You can also have the kids help with creating the décor, which can double up as a fun party activity, and "triple up" as party favors that you can send back home with guests when they are done. Find a thematic art project for them to do, such as decorating a pot to plant a tree in, and use recycled materials and nontoxic art supplies. This keeps kids entertained for a little while, creates decorations onsite that can become a part of any party theme, saves money over other store-bought games, eliminates the need to buy extra party favors, and is less burdensome on the environment.

Simply put, it doesn't take all the trash in the world to make it a great birthday; it just takes a little imagination.

Hey kids! Want to have fun and learn about being nice to animals? Check out this list of party games that will entertain and inform (and quite possibly terrify) all at the same time. These are variations on old party favorites that most parents grew up playing—but with a vegan spin. Bonus: these games are sure to steer (or scare) a few parents toward veganism:

Duck Duck Goose: The object of this game is to walk in a circle, tapping each player's head and saying "duck." When you're ready to choose the next person, say "goose," and the chosen player must chase the picker around a the circle to avoid becoming the next picker. This vegan version includes feeding kids cake through a funnel instead of tapping them on the head. This teaches them indulgence as well as what happens in the production of foie gras.

Pin the Tale on the Piggy: The pork industry's rationale for tail docking is that pigs bite each other's tails, and the tails can then become infected. Of course, they choose to chop the tails off the piglets without anesthesia. Poor piggies. Time to put the tails back on the pigs! This is the same setup as Pin the Tail on the Donkey; just replace the donkey with a pig and use a curled-up pipe cleaner for the tail. Fun *and* educational.

Free Willy: You'll need a stuffed orca for this, or dolphin (or any other sea creature that shouldn't be living the rest of their life in an aquarium), and a very small box. Now, ask each child to see if they can fit the orca into the box. See how that little box is no place for that huge whale to live? Play the documentary *Blackfish* in the background.

Animal Scavenger Hunt: You'll need a variety of small plastic animals to play this game and a box of rubber bands. Place the animals in plain sight around the house. Provide each player with a thick rubber band

and ask them to go "on safari." Once they've "tagged" a wild animal, you get to jump out from behind the couch, playing the part of outback police, and arrest them for poaching.

Charades: Write down the names of animals on scrap paper and have the kids take turns acting out the animals without talking. Then throw in guesses like Miley Cyrus or Daniella Monet. When they ask why those names were mentioned, remind them that people are animals, too. The least confused kid who guesses correctly goes next.

Hot Potato: I had to work a potato into a vegan party somehow, and this classic game fit the bill. Players arrange themselves in a circle and toss a small, round object (a tennis ball, an orange, or even a real potato will suffice) to each other while music plays. The player who is holding the "hot potato" when the music stops is out. The game continues until one player is left—that player is the winner! It's more fun using an actual hot potato.

Animal Hide and Seek: This setup is similar to an egg hunt, but you'll be using plastic toy animals. Make a list of all the animals, and then hide them throughout the house. As kids find them, they can check them off the list and collect them in one area. Upon each discovery, you can talk about how each animal should live out the rest of their lives free to roam and frolic and eat and mate. To make it really interesting, add animal names like the West African Black Rhinoceros, Caribbean Monk Seal, and Tasmanian Tiger to the list, but don't hide them. Explain to the children that these are recently extinct wild animals—and that by going vegan they are saving thousands of animals worldwide per year, including those whose habitats are being destroyed for cattle ranches and palm oil.

Guess the Food: This game requires a few plastic bowls and cut-up fruits or vegetables. Each kid has a turn at being blindfolded. They are given a bowl of the fruit or vegetable, and they have to figure out what's in it based first on smell, then touch, and then taste. The winner gets to eat whatever they identified or feed what they don't want to the losers.

All fun *and* educational.

Presents at a birthday party might be more of a challenge since you are not in complete control over what your guests buy or wrap their presents with; however, it's not out of the realm of possibility to gently affect guests by arranging an eco-friendly, compassionate shopping list (like a wedding registry). Or, better yet, enforce a no-outside presents rule for your kid's birthday, which will prevent a house full of forgotten toys the next month. Instead of having the other kids bring presents, have them create wrapping paper as an activity during the party. Supply them with eco/recycled materials and paint and markers. Get another parent to slip off and wrap the gifts you've already bought with their wrapping paper creations.

As for your own presents for your kids, here are some ideas for the best vegan birthday presents for birthdays or holidays:

Fur & Feathers Board Game: Fur & Feathers is a board game that teaches children the importance of being kind to animals (and how our daily choices affect them), without being preachy or negative. Players get to adopt animals from shelters, answer animal fact questions, and order cruelty-free foods at cafés. The first player to rescue one of each of all five animals wins the game.

The Help Yourself Cookbook for Kids: 60 Easy Plant-Based Recipes Kids Can Make to Stay Healthy and Save the Earth by Ruby Roth (Andrews McMeel Publishing): I am a huge Ruby Roth fan (she has written and illustrated some of the most important children's books on veganism, and she'll also do a portrait of your pet if you pay her). This colorful cookbook was made just for little vegan kids.

Herbivore Clothing: This Portland-based vegan shirt and accessories company creates some of the most amazing pieces of wearable art any-where. You can visit them while grabbing vegan eats from Food Fight vegan grocery the next time you're in the Portland International Airport, or you can order online.

Membership to a farm sanctuary: One of those gifts that keeps giving. Take your kids on a trip to any of the more than two hundred farm sanctuaries in the United States to meet the animals they're now helping save.

Organic Edible Finger Paint: Yep, edible paint! And why not? Kids stick paint brushes, crayons, markers, and everything else in their mouths, so this only makes sense The company "We Can Too" made their paints nontoxic, vegan, gluten-free, and edible. They are made in the USA from rice flour, rice cereal, and fruit and vegetable powders.

Soy-based kid-sized crayons: Sixty-four nontoxic, all-natural soy wax crayons in sixteen colors: red, green, blue, egg yolk yellow, black, brown, orange, purple, pink, grass green, sky blue, sunshine yellow, gray, tan, and peach. Our kids love drawing and coloring, and these are a hit every time.

There is also a complete list of vegan books and movies at the back of this book (page 190) that would make excellent gifts for your good little vegan. Finally, there are also many delicious vegan candies and chocolates available to be handed out as party favors for your kids and their friends.

So, there you go! You can now throw a vegan birthday party like a pro. And to think you only have to do this once per year per child for the rest of eternity.

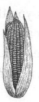

7

THE DOCTOR IS IN: YOUR FAMILY'S CLEAN BILL OF HEALTH

"Children are great imitators. So give them
something great to imitate."
—*Anonymous*

O ne of the most indisputable challenges vegan parents face is
when they take their little ones for regular pediatrician visits
or those "occasional" bumps, bruises, or runny noses. Vegan
kids are in the minority in this setting, as healthcare professionals
aren't always up to speed on the benefits of managing health through
nutrition.

As a side note, Cooper is so athletic (and clumsy) that he has over
one hundred accident reports from daycare, and he used to visit the ER
once a month for a head injury. He's strong enough to lift a Volkswagen
over his head and will dive head-first off any platform or table. He mostly
needs to work on his landings. All the doctors and nurses know him on
a first-name basis. They are pretty impressed that he's in exceptional
physical shape—and that he's vegan. Every nurse, nurse practitioner,

and pediatrician is going to ask you the same set of questions at every visit about your kid's communication level, gross and fine motor skills, problem solving, and, of course, diet. They've all got to be concerned about what your child is eating, right?

Not *entirely*.

Turns out, you may not get all the answers you want or be asked the questions you need from your regular pediatrician. Amazingly, pediatricians may not know much more about nutrition—perhaps the single most powerful driver of your child's health and well-being—than you do. In fact, spend half a day watching the videos on NutritionFacts.org (featuring Dr. Greger), and you *will* know more than they do.

Congratulations, you're now Dr. YouTube.

It's commonly known that nutrition is marginalized in physicians' training. The authors of the book *Nutrition In Pediatrics* wrote that "the teaching of nutrition in medical schools is fragmented at best [and] appears to be entirely unsatisfactory." This report, published in 2006, describes efforts to encourage medical students to consider studying nutrition.

Consider? Studying? Nutrition?

It's actually optional for healthcare professionals to learn about nutrition, otherwise known as the benefits of food for better health. To know that what you put in your body, and in your baby's body, affects their overall well-being and future healthfulness.

The solution touted in the same healthcare report was a discretionary "ten hour workshop." By comparison, the Registered Dietitian (RD) credential requires nine hundred nutrition-specific hours of rotations in hospitals, clinics, and health departments, plus dozens of credit hours in undergraduate and graduate health and nutrition sciences. An RD knows more about the healing power of food than an MD. (For the record, most RDs aren't plant-based. Yet.)

So, what about your pediatrician, the physician who specializes in pediatrics and is concerned with the development, care, and diseases of babies and children? How do we parents broach a vegan diet with our pediatricians (and others); and more specifically, what do we do when they make dietary recommendations like dairy milk for infants?

As we found out in chapter two, Dr. Tom Campbell, who knows a thing or two about what it takes to become a medical doctor, reminds us that pediatricians have been taught that dairy, breast milk from another species, is *essential*. It can often be difficult to address this topic with your pediatrician, but Dr. Campbell offers some strategies to consider when you're trying to get answers from your doctor about nutrition:

- Emphasize that you're trying to get *more* of X,Y, or Z for your kid (fiber, fruits and vegetables, vitamins, etc.). This will provide them with something to focus on and help with in regard to nutrition, and it will show them that you care about what you're putting into your baby.

- Feel free to describe what you eat in specific terms. A physician sitting across the room can be suspicious of the parents who appear to be feeding their kids supposed "vegan" diets, but who are actually starving them with some bizarre nutrition plan. We've all heard the horror stories of parents who had "intuitions" that their infant was allergic to different foods and needed to be gluten-free and could only eat almond milk and walnuts. Tragically, some of those kids end up dying or nearly dying. Offer your pediatrician reassurance that you aren't *that* parent. Your confidence (and persistence) is key.

- Be open to the pediatrician's suggestions and certainly listen to any concerns. They know an awful lot, and you should respect that. Well-fed kids can still have medical problems, so whatever you do, don't fully turn your back on Western medicine. Suggest getting blood tests, if that's a concern. It's not unreasonable to check a B12 level, a metabolic panel, or even just a hematocrit (which is often done with a lead test and is related to potential iron deficiency anemia).

- Follow up with regular office visits according to schedule, if only to check in on your child's growth and development and let the doctor know that everything is going great.

We've had nothing but incredible visits to the doctor with our two toddlers. Their regular check-ups and the occasional unplanned visit (because: Cooper) reassures us that our two vegan babies are thriving.

Need more proof?

Truly, vegan kids are the healthiest kids. J. D. Goldschmidt is a New York City–based actor, model, and personal trainer. His wife and four-year-old daughter thrive on a plant-based diet. His family has been vegan for over two years.

"I stumbled upon a few slaughter house videos and couldn't believe it was real," J. D. says "I went home that night and showed them to my wife, and we decided to be vegetarian. We kept doing a lot of research, and not too long after going vegetarian, we discovered that the dairy industry was just as bad, if not worse, than the meat industry. So, we went vegan. Mia was just under two; she's four now. It's been over two years, and we feel amazing—we have tons of energy, our skin has cleared up, we've gotten stronger in the gym, and we both feel closer to nature."

"I was raised in central Pennsylvania and never even heard the word vegan until I was around twenty-five. You know what they say: 'I could never go vegan,' said every vegan before going vegan."

J. D. is the model of great health and manages to maintain a physique that men want and women notice; or the other way around. He and his wife are seeing the same commitment to fitness in their young daughter, and they know that raising her vegan is giving her the best head start on physical fitness.

"My daughter is definitely into fitness without actually knowing it," J. D. says. "My wife works out at home a lot. We have a pull-up bar in the bedroom, and my daughter naturally joins in. She'll grip the pull-up bar and I'll lift her up and down. She'll do bodyweight squats and jumping jacks with my wife while she's working out. It's fun for her, like a game. She'll even hit a yoga pose or two. It's good we had her young because she has more energy than any person I know; it's hard to keep up with her. She keeps us in shape."

Some of it may be genetics, but I can tell you that with our two toddlers, it's all pure unbridled energy that's powered by plants. Cooper and Paisley pop out of bed at 5:30 a.m. and, literally, keep moving until they crash at 8:30 p.m. It's as if they've been loaded into a slingshot and fired across the planet. Meanwhile, this "planet" is a two-bedroom apartment, and there are a ton of toys and other obstacles in their way along their erratic paths.

Children learn by example. They become little versions of their parents in every way (which also explains why our kids know some "colorful" words, and it's hard not to laugh when they repeat them). J. D. and his wife have set a high bar for physical fitness, and their daughter is taking their lead.

"For my workouts, I stay pretty old school," J. D. says. "I'm a big fan of the classic physique (Steve Reeves, Frank Zane), so I do a lot of compound exercises like incline dumbbell presses, military presses, deadlifts, and squats. I go pretty heavy with these movements and do around four to five sets of each and keep my rep range around six to ten reps per set. I stay lighter on the isolated movements like bicep curls, tricep extensions, leg extensions, and lateral raises and will usually aim for three to five sets, with anywhere from ten to twenty reps to really get the blood flowing."

And his daughter mimics this level of activity *and* diet.

"We follow a high-carbohydrate, moderate-fat, moderate-protein diet. Our diet is made up of 60 to 70 percent carbs, 15 to 20 percent calories from fat, and 15 to 20 percent calories from protein. The majority of our diet consists of oats, potatoes, sweet potatoes, brown rice, quinoa, buckwheat, whole wheat pasta, lentils, beans, tofu, tempeh, seitan, nutritional yeast, nut butters, hemp seeds, flaxseeds, chia seeds, tons of leafy greens, and other vegetables and fruit. We will occasionally have some mock meat products; our favorites are from a brand called Gardein."

Here is another example of a vegan eating grass and sprouts and lacking the protein and required nutrients to be healthy—as some believe. J. D.'s family eats healthy to stay healthy, while still allowing themselves indulgences.

"We will splurge on vegan pizza, vegan ice cream, vegan doughnuts, and stuff like that. Our daughter is definitely not deprived of any treats. My wife is also an amazing baker. She makes healthy muffins and brownies made from black beans, chocolate fudge, cakes, and other treats. Our daughter eats the exact same way we do. A typical day of eating for our daughter would be overnight oats for breakfast, which includes oats, soy milk, cacao powder, hemp seeds, flax seeds, and cinnamon, with a little blackstrap molasses and maple syrup to sweeten it up. For lunch, we have something like a hummus and avocado sandwich on Ezekiel bread, with some broccoli. Dinner would be vegan mac and cheese, using brown rice quinoa pasta, and spinach or some other kind of vegetable. Our snacks are dried fruit, fresh fruit, veggies in hummus or guacamole, crackers, Lara bars, and more."

What advice does J. D. offer to curious parents wanting to raise their own physically fit vegan kids?

"Read books, watch videos by (plant-based) doctors, read peer-reviewed studies. Your child's health is nothing to take lightly. Don't let family or peers pressure you into not raising your child vegan because they think your baby won't get enough nutrients or something. They are misinformed, like the other 99 percent of the world. Study after study shows that a whole food, plant-based diet is the healthiest way to go. If you don't believe me, look up doctors like Michael Greger, Michael Klaper, John McDougall, Neal Barnard, or former president of the American College of Cardiology, Dr. Kim Williams. It is the only diet proven to reverse our number one killer here in the United States—heart disease."

In fact, Dr. Michael Greger warns of heart disease forming in very young children, shockingly before they're even teenagers. By age ten, nearly all kids have fatty streaks in their arteries. This is the first sign of atherosclerosis, the leading cause of death in the United States. The plaques builds in our twenties and gets worse in our thirties; and so on, causes the staggering 1.5 million heart attacks a year in our middle age. Everyone knows someone who has suffered a heart attack, most of which were preventable. In our hearts, these clogged arteries can manifest into a heart attack; in our brains, they become a crippling stroke; in our extremities, it can mean gangrene; and in our aorta, an aneurysm.

Vegans are often referred to as "radical," while preventable open-heart surgery and routine stents are "normal."

So, the question for most of us is not whether we should eat healthy to prevent heart disease, which is the opportunity we have in raising our kids vegan and every reason in and of itself to avoid meat, dairy, and eggs; but rather whether we want to reverse the heart disease we may already have.

True healthcare reform starts in your kitchen, not in Washington, DC.

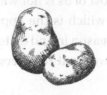

8

A SHOT IN THE ARM: VACCINATIONS AND HERD IMMUNITY

"Mainstream medicine would be way different if they focused
on prevention even half as much as they focused on intervention."
—*Anonymous*

By now, I hope you're convinced that a plant-based diet is the way to go for the optimal health of your kids. You're prepared for anything life will throw your way in regard to your children's health and you know that nutrition is an important part of it all.

Until you read about vaccines.

Let's start here: *no vaccine is vegan.* In fact, there are no prescription or over-the-counter drugs available *anywhere* that are vegan. At some point, the vaccination or drug you need to take has either been tested on animals or contains animal by-products. It's for this reason alone that thriving on a plant-based diet is more important than ever. Most drugs can be eliminated completely by eating healthy, and a whole-foods, plant-based diet is the best prevention for many health issues, which may mean you will never need to be on prescribed medicine, ever.

Seaweed, fruits, vegetables, grains, and whole foods can help you stay healthy and actually heal many symptoms and reverse countless conditions. But what do vegans do when the subject of vaccinations is inevitably broached by your peers, physicians, and well-intended family members?

You vaccinate.

I asked my wife, Jen, to provide her insight into this subject. She is the one who brought the "anti-vaxxer" movement to my attention, and this is her response to the vegan community. I couldn't have said it better myself.

Most vegans I know are introspective and give deep, meaningful thought to how their actions and choices affect others and our planet. Most vegans I know think critically about social, political, and economic disparities. Most vegans I know are trying to live an ethical and moral life and help others along the way. Most vegans I know are concerned about the health and well-being of themselves and their loved ones. Most vegans I know are nonviolent folks who wouldn't want to permanently and severely damage or kill other people, including innocent babies.

Most vegans I know wouldn't drink and drive, endangering their lives and others, even though it's their personal choice to drink. Most vegans I know have a visceral reaction to the unnecessary suffering of animals and also don't like the thought of seeing their fellow humans suffer. Most vegans I know wouldn't visit an oncology ward with even a head cold knowing a simple cold to someone with a compromised immune system could give them pneumonia. Most vegans I know don't exercise their constitutional right to bear arms, thereby making it impossible for them to accidentally shoot other people, even though it would be their personal choice to own a gun. Most vegans I know are loving and compassionate, and I'm fortunate to have them in my life.

Most vegans I know are anti-vaxxers because vaccines are not vegan.

And yet, it is indisputably the fault of anti-vaxxers that we are seeing a serious, highly contagious, and potentially deadly disease reemerge in this country of wealth and privilege and education and freedom. Most vegans I know, my friends, wouldn't want my baby to suffer brain damage or blindness or deafness or even death. Yet their very presence in a room with my daughter could kill her. Most vegans I know want to do the right thing for themselves, their families, and their friends, and for the good of public health.

Most vegans I know strive for an organic lifestyle free of toxins, yet most vegans I know breathe air (polluted with toxins), drink water (polluted with sterilizing chemicals), eat out at nonorganic restaurants, touch plastics, wear nonorganic cotton, buy clothes and use iPhones and droids and computers made halfway around the world in sweatshops, use unsustainable energy, drive cars, fly in airplanes, and generally leave a carbon footprint every day despite recycling efforts, water conservation, and being vegan. Most vegans I know believe in the science of climate change, the science of nutrition, and science in general, but they choose to deny the science of vaccines. Most vegans I know aren't perfect people, but they're doing the best they can.

Please, vegans, vaccinate your kids. Save lives. Do what you say you are all about: compassion, nonviolence, and love for all living beings, which includes doing your part to not kill babies and those who cannot get vaccinated because of weakened immune systems. Your emotional politics are making people suffer unnecessarily, and we will start seeing deaths in this country as a direct result of your inaction. The time to vaccinate is now. You won't be any less vegan, less pure, or less organic for doing so. We can save lives together while at the same time advocating for veganism.

The main reason to vaccinate is because vaccines will protect against severe infectious diseases, dramatically lowering the risk of dying or getting disabled from them. When was the last time you had to think about getting your child fitted for an iron lung?

"Sophie, stay away from Jackson or you might catch polio."

"But, Mom!"

"Don't you 'but, Mom' me . . . isn't it bad enough you're forever trapped indoors, living inside a negative pressure ventilator?"

"You're mean!"

"You're grounded!"

Some of us reject vaccines because we're not convinced they work as advertised or we believe they may have unacceptable side effects. We also reject vaccines solely because they are made from, or tested on, animals. However, wouldn't that seem to lead logically to rejecting most of Western medicine as well?

The people around you rely on your better judgement to contribute to what's referred to as "herd immunity." The more people who cannot contract smallpox means there are less people contracting smallpox. Maybe you will survive a disease that is possible to vaccinate against, but someone who has gone through chemotherapy or a newborn baby who cannot be protected before the age of one might not. If the population is vaccinated, their risk of being infected due to herd immunity is reduced. Also, vaccinations prevent a large number of illnesses and hospitalizations, which saves and frees up countless of resources that the health care system can then use for diseases that cannot be vaccinated against.

At its peak in the 1940s and 1950s, polio paralyzed or killed over half a million people worldwide every year. Today, polio has been eradicated, with the exception of some very small pockets of people in Pakistan, Afghanistan, and Nigeria. Rotary International is currently working on these regions to eliminate the disease.

It's our responsibility to not only protect our own vegan kids but to also consider the kids around us. Protect your littles as you were protected by your own parents, and please vaccinate your children.

Let food be thy medicine.

It's pretty well-documented that the healing properties of food have been reported throughout history by cultures worldwide. More recently, the case for food as medicine has strengthened with an explosion of clinical research showing specifically what health benefits certain foods can offer and what various nutrients are associated with these benefits.

Studies in the past decade have taken nutritional research beyond protein, carbohydrates, fats, vitamins, and minerals. Many fruits, vegetables, and unprocessed whole foods have beneficial properties for human health. As mentioned earlier, chemicals in plants called phytochemicals have been a specific focus in the past decade, offering benefits such as cancer prevention, cholesterol reduction, and hormone regulation, to name a few.

There is truly a cornucopia of nutritional foods that can be used to heal or regulate health issues for both adults and kids alike. Include a few, or all, of these in your good-eating arsenal:

Basil: Studies suggest that eugenol, a compound in basil, can keep your gut safe from pain, nausea, cramping, or diarrhea by killing off bacteria such as salmonella and listeria. So, whip up a batch of vegan pesto and get rid of your kids' belly aches while they load up on carbs.

Beet root/beet juice: Beets are high in immune-boosting vitamin C, fiber, and essential minerals like potassium (good for healthy nerve and muscle function) and manganese (good for bones, liver, kidneys, and pancreas). They've also been said to help with altitude sickness—for when you bring the kids skiing this winter.

Blueberries: Among the fruits with the highest level of antioxidants, blueberries have been linked to lowering cholesterol, reducing diabetes risk, slowing the aging process, improving motor skills, and supporting urinary and vision health. These, and so many other small tasty fruits, are perfect for little hands to grab onto.

Broccoli: Loaded with vitamins such as A, B6, B9 (folic acid), and K, and minerals such as calcium and potassium, broccoli is continuing to earn top honors as a nutritional superstar. Its unique claim to fame comes from its cancer-fighting properties, activated by phytochemicals indole-3-carbinol and sulforaphane. Amazingly, broccoli isn't as difficult to get your kids to eat as you might imagine (think sautéed in vegan butter). It's well worth the effort.

Cherry juice: Cherry juice, concentrate, extract, and pills are often promoted for a wide variety of benefits. These include reducing joint and muscle pain, improving sleep, reducing high blood pressure, controlling blood sugar, preventing gout, enhancing cognition, and improving overall health and vitality. Pit your cherries with a chopstick (push the pit through the meat) and let your kids dive into a bowl of this messy goodness.

Ginger: Ginger is commonly used to treat various types of "stomach problems," including motion sickness, morning sickness, colic, upset stomach, gas, diarrhea, irritable bowel syndrome (IBS), and nausea. It's perfect for those long car rides or family vacations to a Florida farm sanctuary.

Miso soup: Like chicken soup for your cold, minus the chicken and full of living enzymes, vitamins, minerals, and amino acids. It's basically the power combo of nourishment for your little one's body.

Oranges/orange juice: Of course, vitamin C, most commonly found in citrus fruits, is an antioxidant that can reduce cold symptoms by 23 percent, according to RodaleWellness.com.

Pineapple juice: Pineapple juice is five times more effective than cough syrup, according to a study published in *Der Pharma Chemica*. Pineapples contain bromelain, an enzyme with anti-inflammatory properties that fights infections and kills bacteria. (When juice from fresh pineapples is mixed with a little light rum and coconut milk on ice, it also creates a piña colada cocktail just for you to help you cope with your kid's cold.)

Prunes: 'Nuf said. I think we all know what prunes are good for, and I think we all know how effective they are for the job they set out to accomplish. A little bit (8 oz) of prune juice goes a long way in keeping the bowels happy.

Umeboshi: A salt-pickle plum has a powerful antiseptic effect. It has been used as a natural remedy for food poisoning and other digestive problems for centuries in Japan. Umeboshi is very popular in the macrobiotic community.

Seaweed: Also popular in the macrobiotic community: sea vegetables. Any variety of sea vegetables are very good for you and your little one. They'll make you stronger and improve your overall outlook on life, as evidenced by the size and happiness of manatees. Have you ever seen a sad manatee?

Very popular in Asian culture for their healing powers, sea vegetables aren't really appreciated in North America the way they should be.

My friend, macro chef and co-author of *The Great Life Cookbook* Priscilla Timberlake, mentioned to me the other day that someone needs to remind the vegan community what the macrobiotic community knows so well—that sea vegetables are *incredibly* good for you (and your kids). Priscilla and her husband, Lewis, raised four vegan kids on an entirely plant-based and macrobiotic diet, and they are all the model of excellent health.

Macrobiotic diets are based on the concept of how food relates to Zen Buddhism. The diet attempts to balance the yin and yang elements of food and even cookware. People who eat a macrobiotic diet claim that the forces of earth and life are literally fed to us through our food. Feel the power of your peppers. Harness the potential of your peas. Unleash the potency of parsnips. You can increase iron in your diet by using cast iron pans, and nothing is ever microwaved. Macrobiotic diets reduce the use of animal products, they are centered around eating locally grown foods that are in season wherever possible, and meals are consumed in moderation. You're supposed to count the number of chews it takes before swallowing your pressed salad or millet patties.

It's *very* hippie. And *very* healthy.

But, back to sea vegetables. Packed with vitamins, minerals, and nutrients not found in the same levels as in land vegetables, they add amazing flavors to many dishes. Try smashing chickpeas with a fork and adding some crumbled-up seaweed, and you have instant no-tuna salad. Of course, you'll want to add vegan mayo, but that's far from macro.

Probably the most well-known of sea vegetables would be nori. This is the wrapping found on all vegetable rolls (sushi). We buy it in huge volumes. We always roll a sheet over some warm rice, slice the rolls into one-inch pieces, and dip them into ginger-infused, wheat-free tamari. This is a regular snack in our house as it's easy and fun to make. Of course, you can add avocado, cucumber, and carrots for more flavor and color to make healthy veggie rolls.

Grab a life vest and come aboard for a short tour of sea vegetables. There are other sea vegetables you can use, but these are the ones I have tried or used myself in recipes:

Nori: This is mainly used for California rolls/vegetables rolls. It contains iodine, all the carotenes, calcium, iron, phosphorus, and even vitamin C. Usually sold in sheets and toasted, this is one sea vegetable you've probably already tried. The small to-go packs are always in our baby bag and make for a savory treat.

Wakame: High in protein and calcium, this is what is most likely floating in your miso soup. We use this in a soup recipe. Be warned: when added to boiling water, it expands up to seven times its size—kind of like Seymour in *Little Shop of Horrors*. Remove the wakame from the water, cut into tiny pieces, and put it back in the soup. It provides a beautiful salty taste of the sea.

Kombu: Dark purple in color, this sea vegetable, or kelp, adds iodine, calcium, magnesium, and iron to your dishes. It is called "King of the

Seaweed," even though it doesn't have the distinction of growing seven times its size like its counterpart, wakame.

Dulse: Full of potassium and protein. Dulse can actually be lightly fried in sesame oil for a crunchy topping to a salad or as a snack.

Agar Agar: Flavorless, this is used as a thickening agent in many recipes.

For our own two toddlers, we try to avoid most over-the-counter medicines and only ever give them prescription medication when, well, it's prescribed. Meanwhile, we also look out for them with daily supplements (think Flintstones chewables) to make sure they're getting their RDA of all the vitamins and minerals they need. We've found vegan gummy and hard versions of each and pop one in their mouths each morning before daycare.

9

THE GIVING TREE: LESSONS FROM PETA'S 2016 CUTEST VEGAN KID

> "We live on a blue planet that circles around a ball of fire next to a moon that moves the sea, and you don't believe in miracles?"
> —*Anonymous*

Want further proof that a toddler can become a resounding voice for the animals? Wonder what everything I've been preaching in this book sounds like coming out of someone who is four feet tall? Ever think a second grader would be rapping about going vegan?

Meet VeganEvan.

I did. It was at the Animal Rights 2017 National Conference in Washington, DC, where I had the distinct pleasure of being introduced to PETA's Cutest Vegan Kids Contest winner (2016), VeganEvan. Evan and his mom, Shannon, are both ethical vegans, and meeting them would certainly inspire you to realize that it's not only worthwhile to raise your kids vegan, but it also proves that vegan kids are cool. Years ago, Evan may have been thought of as the outcast in his elementary school because of his veganism; today, he is a celebrity in the vegan and animal rights community, making the rounds in all the conferences and festivals and "hamming up" every photo op he can be a part of.

Dope wardrobe, sunglasses, groupies, and all.

How is someone like Evan's mom sure *her* little superstar is getting enough of what he needs to be healthy? You can start by looking at him and his unbridled (a nonvegan term, but it fits here) energy, as well as his mom, as living examples of a positive vegan lifestyle.

"I haven't eaten meat or sea life in over two decades (since I was one year old), so Evan not consuming meat was not a concern for me at all," Shannon says when I quiz her on raising Evan vegan. "As a matter of fact, I was thrilled when he decided to no longer eat meat at age four. I had done tons of research for basically two thirds of my life, and I was already very confident that leaving meat off his plate would only help him to live a happier, healthier life.

"Once I did some more research, it became quite clear that there was nothing he was missing out on by taking dairy and eggs out of his diet, either. In fact, I quickly learned that, just like meat, dairy and eggs are detrimental to human health. Now, if Evan ate vegan macaroni and cheese and Tofurky dogs for dinner every day, like some kids on the SAD, I'd be concerned about him not getting enough nutrition. However, Evan eats such a variety of different fruits, vegetables, legumes, nuts, seeds, etc., that getting 'enough' nutrition has not really been a concern for us at all. He loves the produce department, and one of the most exciting things for him is when we find a new fruit or vegetable we've never had before. The only thing we have taken precaution with is B12. Evan loves the taste of the 'mykind Organics Vitamin B-12 Spray' and does one spray daily."

There you have it again, living proof that leading a vegan lifestyle for health reasons is an acceptable way to raise kids for optimal well-being. Everyone agrees. Well, almost everyone.

"My mom, on the other hand (Evan's grandma, Lynn), was concerned about him possibly not getting all that he needed on a plant-based diet," Shannon continues. "She had many friends in her ear criticizing and questioning Evan's choice to be vegan at such a young age. For this reason, we have had bloodwork done (even though his pediatrician did not see any need for it). After a full year of being vegan, everything came back perfect. My mom, who has also left meat off of her plate for over twenty years, ended up going vegan about a year after us. Now that she has also done research and seen the proof, she is no longer worried a bit."

So, Evan had the advantage of being raised vegan from a very young age by a parent who knows the benefits of veganism. But how would Shannon approach someone trying to convert a kid already on the SAD to a WFPB diet?

"First of all, I would commend them. I'd recommend getting some awesome books to read, like Ruby Roth's *Vegan is Love*, *V is for Vegan: The ABCs of Being Kind*, and *That's Why We Don't Eat Animals*. I would also recommend watching positive videos of vegan kids on YouTube and Facebook. I would encourage them to be extremely honest with the child. Although I did not raise Evan vegetarian, I never lied to him about what foods were. From the beginning, he ate vegetarian most of the time, except when he was with his dad's family. When we went out to eat, he would also get to choose his meal—from when he was about two years old. I just always told him the truth. For example, if he told me he wanted to order a burger, I would make sure he understood that it was part of a dead cow."

While this approach may seem mean or strange to some, it's precisely what we've done with our little ones. I've gone so far as to be that vegan parent who points out the dead animals in the meat case at our local grocery store. I talk with them about the cruelty of lobster tanks at local restaurants.

I'll point them out: "Dead animal. Dead animal. Dead animal. Dead animal. Potato salad that contains ingredient taken from now dead animals." Believe it or not, our kids actually find it humorous, while also realizing that dead cows, chickens, and pigs are beef, pork, and chicken wings. Essentially, you're telling your kid the truth and pointing out the foods that you're avoiding at the same time.

"I don't believe it is right to feed children the animals they love without them knowing or understanding what they are putting into their mouth and body," Shannon adds. "Another tip to help with the transition is to make it fun by choosing recipes where the child can do a lot of the prep or cooking work—and then enjoy the vegan deliciousness together. If they're too young to go near heat, after you measure your ingredients, kids always love to pour the ingredients in. I'm very fortunate that Evan is the complete opposite of a picky eater, but if you're having a hard time with incorporating lots of fruits and greens, make delicious smoothies!"

Freeze ripe bananas (pro tip: peel them before freezing them; I learned the hard way). The next day, drop a frozen banana, some plant-based sweetened vanilla milk, a scoop of peanut butter, and a squirt of Hershey's chocolate into a blender. Blend on high for one minute. If your kid doesn't consume this immediately and ask for seconds, you may have a bigger challenge trying to get them to eat kale. The total nutritional value of this chocolate-peanut-butter-banana shake? Over twenty-five grams of protein and tons of potassium and iron. Done right, smoothies can become your easy go-to fuel for the kids.

"If you're having a tough time with veggies, nuts, and legumes, they can all be disguised and hidden in many different ways," says Shannon. "For example, you could blend zucchini, yellow squash, mushrooms, cashews, and onions in with a pasta sauce, and they'd never even know they were in there. Most important, teach them facts. Education is the key, and it will help them have confidence and be able to defend themselves down the road."

And how did Shannon broach this diet with Evan's pediatricians?

"Evan and I like to tell the whole world that we are vegan. Despite some stories I've heard, I very confidently told Evan's pediatrician when he decided to go vegetarian at age four and when he became vegan soon after he turned five. I was prepared to defend our lifestyle with facts and figures, but to my surprise, his doctor was totally good with it and had no concerns! Although she is not vegetarian or vegan herself, she acted as if it was a great decision. She did mention the possible B12 deficit and was happy to hear that he gets a daily dose.

"If his pediatrician had a negative reaction and insisted that a vegan lifestyle was not optimal, I would have had to find a new pediatrician.

I think many doctors are coming around, thanks to documentaries like *What the Health* (Netflix), so I think having to worry about the doctors will become less of an issue anyway."

What about other parents and well-intentioned teachers and school officials?

"As far as others are concerned, we are not shy about our plant-based diet and vegan lifestyle," Shannon notes. "Everyone we know personally is aware that we are vegan. We have seen every possible reaction, and that's fine with me. When people get upset about it or have anything negative to say, it creates an opportunity to educate them and hopefully help them to see things in the food industry as they really are. At the very least, just by hearing the word *vegan*, we are planting seeds."

So, how has Evan dealt with his fame and being the spokeskid for vegan kids around the world?

"All Evan wants is for the whole world to go vegan. He understands what is happening to the animals and how unjust it is. He understands how badly we are hurting our planet. In addition to the facts he has learned along the way, he has now watched *What the Health* about five times, and he understands how bad the SAD is for human health as well. He wants to fight for what is right! He is more than happy to be a voice for the voiceless, and he knows that people hear what he has to say. He loves being a co-president and spokesperson for Animal Hero Kids because it gives him so many opportunities to reach more people and help more animals! I'd say he's eating up the fame.

"It doesn't matter if we're in Florida, New York, or Washington, DC; Evan knows that he won't go to a VegFest or any type of vegan event without being recognized and asked to rap by at least a few people. I think it has been very encouraging for him to be shown so much love from vegans all over the country and the world! At the 2016 South Florida VegFest, five girls visiting from Israel came running up to us, saying, 'Oh my! That's VeganEvan! We love him! We watch his videos in Israel! Can we please take pictures with him?' Evan has had so many amazing experiences, and he's had the opportunity to meet so many of his heroes."

But fame only goes so far. Like any kid, Evan can get tempted by the dark side of veganism: vegan junk food. What are the pitfalls and dangers of falling into a vegan junk food trap, if any?

"One of the coolest things about a plant-based diet is that there are *so* many recipes you can make that taste similar to traditional 'junk foods' but that are actually super good for you," Shannon says. "For example, Medjool dates can give a smoothie a chocolatey flavor—and unlike chocolate syrup, they are actually very good for you. Using healthy vegan alternatives that taste 'junky' could really help you to avoid falling into a vegan junk food trap. Also, making food from scratch in general will do the same.

"Even though most Americans on the SAD eat animals and their secretions every single day and at almost every meal, I wouldn't recommend converting to a plant-based diet that mimics an SAD with faux meats. I would say that eating premade products, like Gardein and Tofurky, is fine in moderation. They are certainly much healthier than their animal-based counterparts, and they do tend to be high in protein and other good stuff. I would also say it's alright to have some So Delicious ice cream and Oreos once in a while. Are Oreos healthy? Of course not! We are vegan for everything, but especially for the animals, so we have Oreos as a treat here and there. But I think it's important to eat many whole, real, nutrient-rich, unprocessed foods more often than not."

What's next for Evan, and where should other parents or kids turn when starting out on their vegan path?

"Evan is so proud of being vegan! He decided he wanted to go by 'VeganEvan,' and his artist name that he made for himself is 'Green Rapper VeganEvan.' He introduces himself to people as VeganEvan with the hope that they will start asking some questions.

"Kids today are so fortunate to have many amazing vegan role models. They are strong, talented, and compassionate—vegan bodybuilders, surfers, mixed martial artists, football players, runners, etc. It is so encouraging and empowering to see many amazing athletes, and it makes it awesome to be a vegan kid.

"I said it earlier, but knowledge is power for these kids. It is important that we continue to educate ourselves and our kids so we can more effectively help the animals and the planet. Don't worry about what others will think. Switching to a whole-foods, plant-based diet is the best decision that a person can possibly make for animals, the planet, their own health, and the entire human population. We are on the right side of a socially accepted wrong, and our kids will be proud of us for supporting what is just."

When you commit to raising your kids vegan, you've made a commitment to their future. It's easier than ever to raise them vegan, and there are many informative and interesting activities you can engage them in.

"It is so important to involve the kids with food as much as possible—make smoothies, salads, dips, vegan cheeses, cookies, etc., together," Shannon adds. "Visit farm sanctuaries. Do fun activities with them. Showing the kids what it is that their lifestyle supports is crucial and beneficial—and fun. Get them involved with organizations like Animal Hero Kids, PETA Kids, and peta2, the world's largest youth animal rights group. Participate in kid-friendly demonstrations and events and go to VegFests and vegan events that kids can attend."

The world opens up to those who are open to the world.

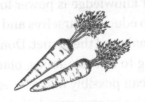

10

TEAMWORK: GETTING THE WHOLE FAMILY ON BOARD

"Teamwork: Simply stated, it is less 'me' and more 'we.'"
—*Anonymous*

Claire and Joe are two vegans whom I got to know through our real-life vegan network. They represent yet another challenge that many families face these days—a blended family. Today the happily vegan couple are the proud parents of three very healthy vegan teens. When Claire and Joe met, Claire brought her son, who has been vegan since birth, into the household, introducing veganism to Joe's two daughters who weren't vegan.

This takes the challenge level of an ordinary blended family and turns up the dial to eleven.

How did Claire introduce the idea of veganism to their older kids?

"Joe and I met when Nicole was nine and a half and Silas and Jessica were both six," Claire tells me during a recent book launch party for *The Skeptical Vegan* she co-hosted at her home. "Silas came with me and has been vegan his whole life. Joe had switched to a vegan diet a few years before we met for health reasons, although he did not immediately have Nicole and Jessica make the switch with him. He slowly introduced them to dairy milk alternatives and tofu, etc.

"When we started dating, Silas and I ate mostly raw vegan, which certainly didn't help bring the girls around to veganism. We ate a variety of salads for almost every meal and went to and hosted many raw vegan family potlucks. The only thing the girls liked about those were the raw desserts."

Raw veganism is a diet that combines the concepts of veganism and raw foodism. It excludes all food and products of animal origin, as well as food cooked at a temperature above 118°F. A raw vegan diet includes raw vegetables and fruits, nuts and nut pastes, grain and legume sprouts, seeds, plant oils, sea vegetables, herbs, mushrooms, and fresh juices. There are many different variations of the diet, including fruitarianism, juicearianism, and sproutarianism. Raw vegans are vegans on overdrive.

Claire knew this would make converting the whole family more work than it might be worth. Selling veganism itself is already a challenge, let alone eating only raw fruits and vegetables. "In order to make our blended family dynamic work, I had to switch back to a plain old cooked vegan diet," Claire confesses.

But trust me when I say that a "plain old cooked vegan diet" in Claire's household is anything but plain. I've been the lucky recipient of some of her amazing vegan meals, and an omnivore wouldn't miss the meat. Claire and Joe hosted our last few ThanksLiving celebrations, and I can personally attest to the fact that no one left hungry.

Claire has been vegetarian since she was nine years old and a strict vegan since she was fourteen based on her ethical view about animal rights. She has worked her entire adult life to help protect animals by educating people about food choices that align with these ideals. Formal courses at the Boulder School of Natural Cookery and the Institute of Integrative Nutrition allowed her to credibly link the benefits of personal food choices to animal welfare.

Claire makes vegan cooking look easy, but blending vegans and omnivores into a new household did pose some challenges, which also extended past the dinner table.

"As one might imagine, Halloween was a bit of an issue for our blended family in the beginning," Claire continues. "Being a pretty militant health nut, Silas had never eaten candy or junk food, and I really did not want him to start. Prior to my marriage with Joe, Silas and I had a group of friends (which included other vegan kids) with whom we would go trick or treating each year. I would make and/or purchase healthier vegan treats in advance and put them in his bag so he could eat along the way.

"He dressed in costume and went to the door with his friends, but unless a toy or vegan chocolate (which does occasionally make an appearance where we live) was offered, Silas did not take it—and he never felt like he was missing out. Nicole and Jessica, however, had already enjoyed traditional "trick or treating" for many years. Joe and I talked about it a bunch before the holiday came up because we wanted to have an agreed-upon plan in place to avoid any argument.

"For our first Halloween together, we decided that Nicole could do her usual trek around our neighborhood with her friends. For Silas and Jess (who were seven at the time), we invited a couple of their friends over and I made treats for them to eat while we watched some Halloween movies. Si and Jess liked it so much that it became a tradition for another two years! A couple of years later, we decided to ban nonvegan candy from Nicole on Halloween.

"She went onto PETA's website, found their vegan candy list, and started trading all of the nonvegan treats (mostly chocolatey stuff) for things like Swedish fish, Airheads, Nerds, etc., with her friends. I held off for as long as I could, disallowing the younger kids from eating candy, but as they reached middle school, we decided it was more important to us that they feel that being vegan is not a hardship, instead of eating healthy all the time. Soon, all three kids referred to PETA's list and began to eat junky, but vegan, candy every Halloween.

"I guess every parent has to make compromises toward their ultimate goal for their children. For me, I want them to want to be vegan for the rest of their lives. I hope that by making certain compromises, it will be an easy choice for them."

Packing lunches for three kids at three different levels of veganism was also something Claire and Joe had to work on together. What did they send their kids off to school with for lunch?

"When Silas was younger, we ate a lot of raw food, so his lunches often consisted of cucumber slice sandwiches or lettuce tacos filled with pesto, nut butter, and hummus, and some fruit and homemade kale chips. Jessica went through a stage where rice or quinoa and beans were her favorite lunch. I often made a lot of baked tofu for the week, which the kids could have in veggie wraps and some sort of cashew sauce or veganaise. They could also have it with veggie sticks and a dipping sauce. Because I have a large family with big appetites, I make very large meals for dinner and often use leftovers for lunches. Stews or stir-fries over quinoa or rice, pasta, chili, etc., all make great lunches."

When it went well, it went well. But there had to be resistance along the way. Luckily for Claire and Joe, their three kids soon came around and ultimately embraced their vegan lifestyle.

"When we married, we decided to put Joe's house on the market, and everyone moved into my house. My raw vegan food business was located in the finished barn, just a few steps from the house. Moving in with me made it easier to make our house an 'all vegan zone.'

"For the first few months, whenever we went out, we let the girls eat whatever they wanted at home. Then, we made meals vegan whenever Joe and I were paying for the food, explaining that we did not want to support animal agriculture. By the end of our first year of marriage, our rule was this: everyone ate vegan when we were together. In other words, the girls could still eat animal products at friend's houses or when staying with relatives.

"After about a year or so, since Jessica was only eight, we decided that we wanted her to be vegan all of the time. Jessica really loves animals, so we took her to a farm sanctuary in Watkins Glen, New York, which helped to solidify her resolve to remain vegan with her family. We explained to her all of the reasons we chose to be vegan, saying that we wanted her to share that with us. She was so close to being all vegan anyway, and fortunately, her friend's parents were very willing to accommodate her diet whenever she visited their homes.

The road to veganism for Nicole was a little different.

"Nicole turned eleven right before Joe and I got married, and she has her own opinions on everything!" Claire exclaims. "She considered veganism as something that hippies did, and she had a very strong dislike of hippies at the time. She also really loved comfort and junk foods, while I was a complete health nut.

"Nicole was always a nervous kid. She did not like to be different in any way, which was a big part of the reason she resisted going vegan. We worked on winning her over with food, rather than forcing it. I went to a wonderful vegan culinary school when I was younger, and one of the many things I learned was how to veganize just about anything.

"I let Nicole help me pick the meals I would make each week to ensure that she would enjoy what she ate. The summer before she started eighth grade, she stayed with her cousins for a couple of weeks, when she ate meat and dairy for the first time in a while. When Nicole came home, she told us that her stomach had felt awful the entire trip from the food she was eating and declared that she had come to the decision to be vegan! We were both excited and surprised that she had made this choice on her own. During this time, it still took her a couple of years before she was willing to even say the word *vegan* among friends.

"If Nicole had friends over, she wanted food that would naturally be vegan but not overly healthy—like falafel, pasta salad, and fries. If she went to friend's houses or parties, she would eat before going because she absolutely did not want anyone to know she was vegan. She learned what to look for in case she got hungry while with friends and would very discreetly check labels on chips before eating them. During the summer of tenth grade, when Nicole went to a five-week summer music camp in Colorado, we called the camp ahead of time to make sure they could accommodate her meals, which they did wonderfully.

"While there, Nicole began to identify herself as vegan for the first time. She was surprised to find that her peers were really impressed, and they dubbed her the 'vegan cutie.' She began to own her veganism. When she visited Boulder, she found that amazing vegan options were everywhere. Her friends ate vegan along with her and complimented her strength and compassion. That trip marked a change in Nicole's confidence, in not just being vegan, but in becoming her own person and showing that person to to the world regardless of what they might think.

"Nicole is a smart, thoughtful, cuddly, and funny vegan band geek who is now about to head off to music school (in Boulder, of all places). She proudly wears funny vegan shirts and Instagrams her vegan food creations with the hashtag #govegan. She finally feels proud of her vegan lifestyle and loves the added benefit of being able to eat delicious food while easily remaining healthy and fit."

"Overall, we try to instill in our children a sense of responsibility to care for our planet and show kindness to all living beings. I truly think this helps them to understand the importance of eating responsibly and living a life that is true to their beliefs."

What's the one tip Claire would tell a parent who is struggling with the day-to-day and school-focused challenges that vegan kids face?

"Be prepared!"

This vegan scout motto has been the resounding theme of the book so far. There used to be a saying among the vegan community that before you're invited out to dinner with friends, you should eat dinner. This way, you go nowhere hungry and won't be disappointed if there aren't vegan options. Though new vegan options are popping up more than ever, this is still somewhat the case. And with kids, it's always good to be prepared.

"If your young child goes to school or daycare, there will most likely be lots of birthday celebrations," Claire adds. "Find (or make) a vegan treat that you child loves and bring it to their school on the first day. You want it to be something that is either shelf-stable or that can be frozen, for example, your child's favorite cookies, ice cream bars or popsicles, homemade truffles, etc. This makes it easy for your child's teacher to grab the vegan option quickly, and your child won't feel left out.

"When traveling, make sure to bring a bag filled with snack foods in case your meals are more spread out. Use Happy Cow (website or app) to find restaurants or stores enroute, and plan your stops according to your food options."

What does the future hold for Claire, Joe, Nicole, Jessica, Silas, and the other 2.5 million vegans in the United States?

"The world is becoming more and more vegan-friendly every day, which will (hopefully) make it much easier for my kids to stay vegan," says Claire. "When I made the switch to a vegan diet in 1994, I was fifteen years old. Hardly anyone knew what the word meant. When I went out to restaurants, my only options were iceberg salads or vinegar and French fries. Mainstream grocery stores carried tofu and maybe hummus, but no other specialty vegan items. Even in health food stores, it was hard to find a veggie burger that did not have eggs in it at the time. It took a very strong will to stay vegan, especially when traveling—which I did a lot of.

"It's amazing how much more accessible vegan specialty products have become over the past twenty-plus years. It's no longer a hardship to maintain a vegan diet and lifestyle. As a fashion lover, I really suffered for years in the shoe department, but now it's hardly an issue—I have a bunch of favorite brands that I can count on, and I come across new brands all the time. Even in the mainstream fashion industry, the term 'vegan leather' has become quite a trend."

In the 2017 film *Bladerunner 2049*, Ryan Gosling set the vegan world on fire when he sported his custom-made vegan leather jacket. There are vegan versions of leather, silk, and wool that are every bit as beautiful and durable as their animal-derived counterparts.

Claire has some final advice about staying vegan in the long term.

"It is important to me that our teenage kids feel like being vegan is something to be proud of, instead of being embarrassed by being different because of the way they eat. This will help them to stay vegan for the rest of their lives. Our house has become the 'hangout' house for the kids and their friends. I make sure to have lots of vegan snacks on hand and fixings for vegan 'junk food' meals that I can make or they can make themselves. Even the friends who were most hesitant about items like vegan cheese now love it! Their friends think it's cool that our kids are vegan, and many have even started asking their parents to buy their favorite vegan products.

"Another thing that has been really wonderful and helpful is that our extended family members have slowly adopted a vegan lifestyle over the years. When Silas, who was my parents' first grandchild, was a baby, I let my family know that it was extremely important to me that they support his vegan lifestyle. That meant not eating meat around him (which

I still think is not such a big thing to ask!). When Silas was younger and we spent the holidays at my parents' home, we discussed in advance and agreed that all of the holiday meals would be vegan, with the exception of some turkey slices that my stepfather bought and kept out of sight.

"My brother, Sean, went vegan when Silas was three years old. My own mother has eaten a mostly vegan diet for many years now. Joe's brother, John, and his wife decided to go vegan shortly after they first started dating and are now raising two healthy vegan children. After years of sharing vegan family meals, our nieces from Joe's brother, Bill, have become vegetarian and are working toward maintaining a completely vegan diet. And when Joe's dad was dealing with a serious heart problem, the brothers showed him the research on vegan diets reversing heart disease. We gave Joe's parents vegan cooking and grocery shopping lessons and lots of vegan cookbooks. Finally, Joe's dad was able to lower his cholesterol to exceptional numbers, as well as becoming more active and fit. He continues to adopt a mostly vegan diet today.

"So, one by one, our family is embracing our lifestyle. Being vegan no longer seems so abnormal for our children."

And being vegan is no longer abnormal for the world.

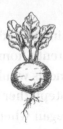

11
ANIMALS ARE NOT FOOD:
WE DON'T EAT OUR FRIENDS

"No act of kindness, no matter how small, is ever wasted."
—*Aesop*

It's a sunny September afternoon in Everytown, America.

Picture a schoolyard filled with happy kids. Blue skies. Birds chirping. The energetic children are bouncing balls, playing catch, sliding down the slides, monkey-barring, wrestling with each other in the grass; all under the watchful eye of their teachers. This is fourth grade recess, and it's among the greatest moments of a young kid's life.

The school playground; where innocence and imagination collide.

Now, imagine a rope being lowered from above into the center of the playground with a frosted vanilla cupcake attached to a noose. It is left dangling in close proximity to the kids. One by one, each child is lured toward the treat as it circles a slow, methodical path around the playground, waiting for the fastest, strongest, and biggest kid to take the bait.

Now, imagine that kid. The fast one. Successfully jumping that extra few inches in the air, he opens his mouth wide, trying to eat the treat. Suddenly, the noose on the rope tightens around his neck as he is immediately dragged upwards. He begins suffocating. Struggling.

The rest of the kids scatter in fear, screaming. The teacher tries to reach the boy, but it's too late. He is being strangled and all the fighting in the world won't release him. He eventually suffocates to death and is skinned and needlessly sautéed for dinner by the person or creature at the other end of the rope.

School's out.

This is the scenario that fish experience when getting caught—pulled from their home, friends, and family. Scoped up into a net and landed into a boat to suffocate. Fish suffer as much as any animal and do not belong in a vegan lifestyle.

No animals are food.

"When we introduced the idea of veganism to our kids when they were, respectively, two and four years old," says Sherry Colb, "we basically told them that we would no longer be consuming dairy and eggs because we would be doing wrong to the animals. One of them asked why it wasn't wrong to the animals the prior week, when we were still eating dairy and eggs. We explained that sometimes we learn that something we were doing before was not right, and we try to do better in the future.

"Introducing animal rights and compassion to the kids was a very positive experience. Unlike other children, who have to be taught to numb themselves to the feelings of the creatures they consume, our kids have had the advantage of getting the unvarnished truth about what most people call food, and we have been able to tell them that their behavior spares numerous animals. It helped a lot when we brought them to their first animal sanctuary because we could then explain that these were the animals they were not hurting."

Children are taught to numb themselves to the feelings of the animals they eat. They know it's not right and not something they would willingly take part in, but parents force their beliefs onto their children that eating animals is good.

Animals are not food.

When our baby girl was born, I made the announcement on social media and fielded the usual questions about raising newborn vegan babies, including the comments about whether breast milk is vegan.

I usually ignore them, but one comment I couldn't ignore was about raising vegan babies in the first place. After all, we had previously fostered twin boys and fed them a vegan diet while they were with us (which, by the way, is its own controversy in dealing with foster kids), and now we had every intention of raising our son and new baby vegan.

The comment said: "Shouldn't your kids be given 'the choice' of whether or not to be vegan?" Obviously, they were trying to stir things up a bit. There are numerous things wrong with what this person was saying:

1. Breastfeeding babies are vegan already, and when they transition to other milk, plant-based milk is better for them than dairy milk (see chapter two).

2. When babies transition to solid foods, the best diet for them is plant-based. Nearly all baby food is made from fruits and vegetables. Think about most of the baby foods out there—most are vegan. Starting a one-year-old on bacon (even bacon that has been pulverized in a blender) is not recommended by most doctors.

3. Babies look to their parents for the best nutrition possible, and there was no way we would put our own child at risk.

As parents, we all naturally make "a choice" for our babies (who can't speak or choose) when we feed them food (vegan or not). Bottom line? Infants don't have (and shouldn't have) choices at a young age. Parents know what's best. Once they become defiant teens, that's a different story.

Giving them a choice to select their diet would be the same as giving them the choice to wear sunscreen or not. Are you going to wait until they can make their own decisions on whether or not to burn themselves to a crisp? No, of course not, you're protecting them from long-term health issues—and that's exactly what a vegan diet does for growing children.

This reminds me of the great *Vegan Sidekick*, a popular online vegan comic strip by Richard Watts. The two-panel strip features a parent holding her little one's hand as she talks to another parent.

First panel:

Person one: "I don't make my child eat meat."

Person two: "Forcing your way of life on your children is extreme."

Second panel:

Person one: "I make my child eat meat."

Person two: "Forcing your way of life on your children is awesome."

Parents need to commit and think through the process of introducing veganism to kids. "I would tell such parents to start with adding things to the menu and then start prohibiting the bad foods later," Colb says. "Make a delicious vegan lasagna or quiche with Follow Your Heart's VeganEgg. Bake great desserts using vegan recipes from Vegweb.com. Once the kids see that the food is great, they'll have an easier time 'giving up' the animal-based foods that they believe they must have."

Some parents may feel inconvenienced, in spite of the fact that everything they've chosen to eat in the past has a vegan version waiting to be tasted. As I quoted Colb back in the introduction: "A lot of the inconveniences of veganism turn out to be that, an inconvenience of having to find our way through a nonvegan world.

"The vegan movement can learn from the disability rights movement," Colb adds. "Disability rights activists have long argued that the very idea of 'disability' is social. For example, before curb cuts were common, people in wheelchairs had much greater difficulty navigating sidewalks and streets, but that was not because wheels are inherently inferior to legs; it was because the streets and sidewalks had been designed based on the assumption that everyone locomotes with legs. Likewise, eating vegan at unfamiliar restaurants is only a challenge when the restaurant owners have assumed that very few of their customers are vegan."

I was tweeting the other day—vegans are known to tweet up to five times a day due to the amount of *fiber* (optics) in our diet—and I came across this headline: "Dolphin Safe Does Not Mean Tuna Safe," and it made me think about how often consumers are often duped when shopping for food. They are somehow led to believe that their choices in what they purchase and consume is okay based entirely on marketing terms.

In this case, who is looking out for the tuna? Or, the other 250,000 species of marine life that are captured and killed for food? And while the dolphin may be "safe" from this one company (they aren't), they are hardly safe from the other human horrors they face every day in their waters, not the least of which is pollution (which is associated with the meat and dairy industries).

"Free-range" and "grass-fed" are two other examples of catchy marketing slogans to make omnivores feel better about what they're buying. In whatever ways the animal is treated in advance of being caged, tortured, and killed makes little difference to the animal. Of course, animals can't read (although some chimpanzees can use typewriters and understand sign language). For the meat eater, these words might make a difference, but it's not much of a consolation to the chickens, pigs, turkeys, and cows they are referring to.

"Cage Free" indicates that birds are raised without cages, but it does not describe other living conditions. Cage-free eggs could have come from birds raised indoors, in overcrowded conditions, and without access to daylight, let alone pasture. The USDA has not developed any standards for this label, and it, along with other yuppy marketing terms, is misleading to the consumer. If someone witnessed the treatment and conditions a "cage free" hen is legally allowed to endure, I don't think they'd buy eggs anymore.

Basically, if the carton says "cage," those hens aren't free.

"Animal Welfare Approved" means the animals have access to the outdoors and are able to engage in natural behaviors. No cages or crates may be used to confine the animals, and growth hormones and sub-therapeutic antibiotics are not allowed. Some surgical mutilations, such as beak-mutilation of egg-laying hens, are prohibited, but others, such as castration without anesthesia, are permitted. Not sure if you've ever seen videos of how farmers castrate baby pigs, but this act alone is enough for me to say I am vegan for life.

There is a belief that "hormone-free" milk is much better for you than any other kind of milk . . . you know, the kind that contains casein, the cancer-escalating phosphoproteins. It isn't. There is a reason milk marketing doesn't mention casein. No one would ever buy milk again (which would be quite a relief to those hormone-free, grass-fed, raped-by-a-farmer dairy cows). By the way, all milk has hormones.

Probably the most troubling of these labels is the one so many boutique butcheries brag about in their marketing: "Humanely Slaughtered." There is nothing humane, ever, about killing someone who doesn't want to be killed. Although the United States technically has "humane slaughter" laws, they provide very little protection to pigs, cows, sheep, and goats and do not provide *any* protection for chickens, turkeys, or other birds.

Maybe one day the ridiculousness of all this labeling will reach its apex with the rollout of labeling on meat, dairy, and egg products that reads: "Just Murdered." And when consumers still choose to purchase these products, then we'll know there is little hope left for society.

Alex Hershaft is the founding president of Farm Animal Rights Movement (FARM), arguably the oldest animal rights organization in the country. His own life experience, having survived Auschwitz and the Warsaw ghetto, led to a lifelong mission to save the animals, and he founded FARM in 1977. Through innovative programs that reach young minds with animal rights advocacy and messaging, Alex may be personally responsible for converting thousands toward veganism over the span of his career.

He also happens to be my boss.

"Well-meaning folks have challenged my decision to devote the rest of my life to promoting animal rights and fighting all forms of oppression, especially our oppression of animals raised for food," Hershaft says. "Why animals, they question, when so many human problems remain unsolved?

"Because oppressing animals is the gateway drug to oppressing humans. When we tell a child that the family dog on his couch is to be loved and cherished but the pig on his plate is to be tortured, slaughtered, dismembered, and consumed as food; that society can arbitrarily decree that one sentient living being can live, but another must die, we plant the first seeds of discrimination and oppression against *all* beings.

"Why animals? Because they are an integral part of our fondest childhood memories. Toy animals were the very first objects we handled. Our favorite fairy tales revolved around animal lives. Our family dog gave us unconditional love, when our schoolmates or even our siblings would not. Walt Disney and others made a fortune bringing back those cherished memories. It was only the greed and insensitivity of the meat and dairy industries that turned our favorite living beings into a commodity to be exploited and oppressed."

Why animals? Would you tell your kids that Porky Pig is where bacon comes from? Or that sushi is made out of Nemo? Or that you had Donald Duck confit at your anniversary dinner? Or what would your kids think about Bambi kabobs on the barbecue?

Who ate Roger Rabbit?

Keith Allison is a licensed educator in the state of Ohio, where he lives with his three boys, Brady, Spencer, and Elliott. He enjoys speaking with students and watching their minds explore new concepts. He is an avid film geek and enjoys hiking, biking, swimming, and spending time with his family and friends. And he is an animal rights activist.

Keith made national news in 2015 when he won a free speech legal battle against the Green Local School District, in Green, Ohio. He had previously lost his job as a teacher because he chose to shed light on a subject the school district wanted to keep hidden. Keith's incredible story is a reminder to all that standing up is as powerful as taking a knee.

Teaching kindness, compassion, and respect for life should be among the most valued lessons we find inside a school. It is astonishing to me that we don't always value and nurture those qualities in our children. Instead, we often teach them to distance themselves from feelings they already have. Too often, when confronted with our children's compassion in the face of the realities of our current society, we tell our children to "toughen up" or "grow up," or that it is "just the way things are." We tell them it is "necessary" even when it isn't. Teaching a child to be kind to a dog but to bite into a pig is a strange lesson that conflicts with our values of compassion and kindness. We should, inside a school, be teaching them to critically examine concepts even when they don't align with the status quo. But when it comes to questioning the idea of killing animals for our food, too often we don't want discussion. We want silent acceptance of social norms.

What got me removed from my teaching job, however, had nothing to do with what I taught my students. My job was taken away because of what I posted on Facebook to my friends, outside of school property and on my own computer.

As a Title I teacher, I led small group instruction for children needing a little extra help in math or reading. I had fun interacting with great kids as we worked on improving their understanding of things like fractions and reading comprehension. I wasn't a vegan activist while on the job; I was a *teacher*.

Outside of my job, however, I have my own voice and speak up for what is important to me. One day, as I was biking along, not far from home, I came across rows of calf crates. The separation of babies from their mothers in the dairy industry is one of the darker sides of agriculture that are often kept hidden from the public, but these crates weren't hidden. They were perfectly visible just off the road, on the side of the driveway. I couldn't shake that image as I finished biking home, so I returned by car, stopped on the road, and took a quick picture from my car.

In spite of almost universal public opposition, hundreds of thousands of calves (the male offspring of dairy cows) who are raised for veal are intensively confined in individual plastic crates too narrow for them to even turn around. Tethered to further restrict any movement, they're virtually immobilized for their entire sixteen-week lives. Unfortunately, this confinement is common in the veal industry, despite overwhelming scientific evidence that it's inhumane, and most people outside the industry oppose it. Keith continues:

If we are going to consume animal products, it is time we are honest about them. Cows do not "give" milk to humans. We take it. We impregnate cows so they will produce milk (something all mammals do to nourish their babies), and once their baby is born, we take the baby so we can drink the milk instead. This is not a gift to us from a cow. Cows don't willingly break the mother-child bond. They don't think humans having milkshakes is more important than their baby being fed. Humans decide our desire for cheese is more important than a calf's desire and need to be with her mother, to have food, or to even have life. And then we have the audacity to teach our children that these are "happy cows giving milk." Reality has been distorted, intentionally hidden from view. I wanted to bring it back into view.

Without naming the farm, I posted a close-up picture of these crates on my Facebook page, with the following caption:

This place is five miles from my house, and, for those who don't already know, these are crates to house baby dairy cows who are separated from their mothers usually within a day of birth. As someone who grew up feeling parental love and support, and now as a parent who gives parental love and support, I reject the claim that separating babies from loving mothers to raise them isolated in boxes can ever be considered humane.

In the comments, I added, "The cruelty of separation, loneliness, and infant slaughter lingers inside each glass of cow's milk. Your voice can help change the system. You don't have to support this. Plant-based milks are everywhere and are delicious."

I really didn't expect much. That's what happens on Facebook. A few sympathetic friends might like the post or comment with a crying emoji. Maybe it would give a few others something to consider. I never expected anything beyond that.

What I did receive was a meeting with my superintendent after the second day of school. As the Title 1 teaching positions were all one-year contracts and my verbal rehire came shortly before the start of the year, the board of education had yet to officially approve my contract when the year began. My superintendent had received a phone call from the farmer the day of the board meeting. Concerned by the complaint, the superintendent pulled my name from the board meeting so I did not get the opportunity for approval. I was retroactively changed into a substitute teacher while she "looked into things." I was threatened with a written reprimand and sternly advised that if I wanted to continue to be a vegan activist, I might want to consider doing something other than teaching. By the end of the week, I was unemployed.

I waited patiently, thinking things would be resolved and I would be reinstated. Parents, upon learning I was gone, were voicing their displeasure with my removal. When it became apparent that the school would not reconsider, I began exploring my options and found legal representation through the ACLU of Ohio. On December 10, 2014, my attorney, Joseph Mead, sent a demand letter to the school citing violations of my first amendment rights. It stated, among other things, "Urging people to drink soy milk on Facebook is not a fireable offense." The demand letter insisted on a prompt apology, reinstatement of my employment, back pay, and attorney's fees.

Driven by the first amendment angle, this public demand letter drew widespread interest. News organizations, both local and international, wanted to learn more about and report on this story in small-town Ohio. In the midst of the media coverage, but not part of any settlement, the school offered me a position similar to the one from which I was removed. I returned to work in January, but no true efforts were made to remedy the loss of income during the time I was wrongly terminated nor reimburse my attorney fees.

We filed a lawsuit against the school district on March 4, 2015 and settled the case on April 13. I received full back pay and attorney's fees. While I never received the apology, the school district did acknowledge within the settlement agreement that "Green Local Schools recognizes the rights of its staff members, within the confines of the law, to engage in free speech outside the educational setting."

No teacher should lose their voice. We don't sign away our individual rights by stepping into a classroom. Outside of school grounds, we are still citizens, and part of our responsibility as citizens—of this country and this world—is to strive to improve it. We can't accomplish this if our mouths are closed in fear of retaliation. Blindly following the status quo has never brought about change. True change—and with it, true progress—only happens when we are willing to speak out.

With help from the ACLU and the PETA Foundation, Keith is now back at work teaching at a different school in the district, and he remains a field educator for Ethical Choices Program.

Every moment is a teachable moment. And little by little, a little becomes a lot.

Nathan Runkle is an American animal rights advocate and the founder and executive director of Mercy for Animals, an international nonprofit organization dedicated to preventing cruelty to farmed animals and promoting compassionate food choices and policies. Mercy for Animals was founded in 1999, when Nathan was just fifteen.

Today, Mercy for Animals has an annual operating budget of nearly twelve million dollars. In 2016, it distributed 1.5 million pro-vegan leaflets and captured 1.7 million vegan pledges.

I had the pleasure of meeting Nathan at the Animal Rights 2017 National Conference and hearing him speak. His story is truly inspiring. This was in August, a month before the release of his own first book, *Mercy for Animals*.

Of all the stories you might read or hear as you explore raising your kids vegan, Nathan's story may resonate the most as he began his own journey to veganism at such a young age. Nathan is who we hope our own kids become when we set out to raise compassionate humans. Perhaps one day our young vegans, too, will go on to accomplish incredible things for the movement. Nathan says:

Eating animals does not come naturally to any child. Our initial instinct is kindness, not cruelty. I saw this play out dramatically during my own childhood in rural Ohio. Most kids were 4-H members. In these programs, they learned to raise farmed animals. I'd watch my peers grow attached to their friends, tenderly bottle-feeding the calves and piglets. As the county fair approached, the kids were devastated to learn the fate of their companions—slaughter. I remember children wailing, their arms thrown around their doomed friends' necks. Over the years, I saw these same kids become hardened and detached.

When we raise children to eat animals, we teach them to disconnect from their natural empathy. We also impart one of the most damaging lessons a person can learn: that one group can be inferior to another simply because they are different. In this case, that group is animals, but the ripple effects of this rationalization are felt throughout our society in the forms of racism, sexism, classism, homophobia, and every type of discrimination based on a might-makes-right belief.

When we raise children vegan, we teach them that compassion should extend to everyone, regardless of their vulnerability. They learn that bullying is wrong, to respect other bodies, and that something isn't right just because everyone is doing it. We raise them on a diet that is healthier not only for their growing bodies but for their moral development.

Some parents worry that their children will have to deal with feeling "different." I can tell you that, at least in my case, going vegan at such a young age only made me a more successful, thriving young adult. I started Mercy for Animals when I was just fifteen years old, and I was able to do so because I'd been practicing making the ethical choice for years.

Three times a day, we have a choice. Let's choose to teach our children compassion with every meal and help build a brighter future for all of us.

Kindness is contagious.

12

LUNCH LADY LAND: HOLD THE STEAMED CHEESEBURGER

"The belly rules the mind."
—Spanish Proverb

Whether your kids are homeschooled or in daycare, elementary school, middle school, high school, or college, they've got to eat. I can say firsthand that our own kids make a beeline for the fridge and the pantry the moment they come careening in the front door, dangling off the door like Tarzan, yelling, "I need food!"

No matter what grade they are in, they're going to have to face certain challenges in each phase of their academic life if they are vegan. Not the least of which is the fact that crayons aren't vegan but Elmer's glue is. Go figure. Neither of these items should be considered food, but nonetheless they still end up inside our toddlers.

You can rely on the foods provided in the school cafeterias and dining halls or you can pack their lunches. Of course, packing lunches gets awkward by the time you've sent them off to college, so you might want to be better prepared and get involved in what they're eating at school sooner rather than later.

School lunches are notoriously terrible and limiting (although the situation is improving). As a concerned parent, you need to know if there is anything you can do to encourage your daycare or school to offer more vegan and plant-based options. For the record, seeking "vegetarian" options at school isn't really as meaningful as it might sound, since that would include gooey cheese dripping off greasy pizza.

"Families, parents, and kids have most of the control when it comes to changing the school lunch line," Dr. Neal Barnard says. "Don't be shy, and voice your opinion to the food service staff, principal, teachers, superintendent, and school board. The Physician's Committee for Responsible Medicine (PCRM) has lots of resources to help with these endeavors. Check out HealthySchoolLunches.org for more information."

And what kinds of food can we send them off to school with?

"So many lunches that children enjoy are already vegan," Dr. Barnard adds. "The classic peanut butter and jelly sandwich is always a hit. Cubed and slightly browned tofu makes a tasty entree, and its nutrient content and wholesomeness far surpasses something like a chicken nugget. Snacks like pretzels or whole-grain crackers are a great accompaniment. A serving of fruit is sure to please—strawberries, grapes, and apple slices. Depending on the child's age, cut the sandwich or fruit into small pieces so they are easy to eat."

In our household, we send our kids off with either a vegan cheese sandwich or peanut butter and jelly with cut up fruit, crunchy veggies, and maybe a snack bag of granola or chips. They're also provided vegan snacks and nondairy milks by the facility.

Amie Hamlin is the Executive Director of the Coalition for Healthy School Food (CHSF), an organization dedicated to changing menus in schools across New York State (and beyond). Their website, HealthySchoolFood.org, offers a wealth of information on this subject, as does Amie. She also happens to be a close friend of mine, and I can tell you that she is as passionate a vegan as you'll ever find.

The Coalition for Healthy School Food (CHSF) is a nonprofit organization that introduces plant-based (vegan) foods and nutrition education in schools to educate the whole school community— kids, parents, teachers, paraprofessionals, administrators, other staff, and food service professionals. They do this by developing from-scratch vegan menu options to replace meat, eggs, and cheese. Working with companies that manufacture clean vegan foods, CHSF targets PreK-12 food service directors to get vegan foods items on the menus and creates materials and resources to promote these vegan options for school-aged kids. While based in New York State, their vegan recipes have been distributed to 25,000 schools nationwide, and some of their resources reach tens of thousands of students every day. In addition, they will help any school in the country who needs help.

Everything plant-based starts with a seed. And, from there?

"Always have food *for* your child," Amie says. "This is true for class parties, school field trips, after-school programming, and sports."

So, what does Amie send her own high-school-aged daughter, who is both vegan and gluten-free, off to school with each day?

"At this point, she makes her own food. Basically, PB&J, fruit, cut up veggies. Nothing too exciting. She likes the basics." Which is always a good place to start with anything, especially when sending kids off with vegan food. Begin with the essentials and build up from there as your child starts to experiment with more adventurous plant-based fare.

Even though we want our kids to eat healthy—and they should the majority of the time—you should also give them special treats from time to time: ice cream, candy, cookies, cake. They are already different enough from other kids with a restricted diet, and you don't want your child sneaking behind your back when they can't have the equivalent of what other kids have. All that said, I totally respect it when parents choose not to give their children these foods.

"You can make truly healthy homemade special treats," says Amie. "But if you are okay with some vegan junk foods, send your child with a special treat (something they don't normally get) so they feel like they are not deprived relative to the rest of the kids. Oftentimes at school, these things came up and my child returned home upset because everyone else had something special and she didn't. So I made cupcakes and had the school put them in the freezer, labeled for her. The teacher would get one out on days when there was a celebration to thaw it out in time.

"Also, we were lucky because her school always purchased nondairy ice cream to accommodate her and others. That said, I would have preferred that she wasn't getting that stuff at school. Another option is for your younger child to do a presentation in school about why they eat this way and bring special treats for all the other kids. Present it to the teacher as diversity, because it *is* a type of diversity."

Most challenges are surmountable. Some are easier than others, but some we wish we never had to deal with.

"My daughter was bullied for her veganism in school, and that was serious. It had an impact on her," Amie says. "I did not realize what was going on and I thought the school had dealt with it. By the time I realized the extent of it and she was able to verbalize it to me, I spoke *again* to the school, but she was already going into a new grade. That teacher did label it as bullying, which I did prior to that (and the previous teachers did not agree with that label for what was going on, too). Luckily, the new teacher dealt with it and the problem ended. But to this day, my daughter is unhappy if she ever runs into that child, who interestingly, has a vegetarian father.

"The takeaway message is to be very aware that this is a possibility and to have discussions with the teacher and your child to ask if anything is going on. Our children can often answer a question such as 'What do other kids say about what you eat?' but they may not be able to approach you to say that a child is bothering them. Let the teacher know that your diet and lifestyle is a deeply held ethical belief. Tell them that you know that children are sometimes made fun of or bullied for it, and that it is very important to you that the teacher be aware of this. Ensure that they keep their eyes open and deal with it *and* let you know if they see anything going on."

Now, what if you are interested in working with what is served in school cafeterias?

Schools are often dictated what they can and cannot serve based on antiquated FDA guidelines for nutrition. Sometimes these foods are subsidized so much, making them much more affordable and leaving schools with no choice but to serve them to students.

This is the case with dairy.

"Milk is another issue. School cafeterias are plastered with milk posters. Growing up, many of us learned that milk builds strong bones. But you might have noticed that while the dairy industry no longer claims that milk builds strong bones, the posters and milk ads continue to say that milk has protein, potassium, and calcium, showing little kids next to big football players and celebrities and continuing the myth. What message are they trying to give our kids?

"While there is no requirement to serve meat or cheese, milk must be offered (it does not need to be consumed, contrary to popular belief). It would literally take an act of Congress to change this requirement. Given that milk is a *probable* carcinogen for prostate cancer, a *possible* carcinogen for ovarian cancer, mildly associated with teen acne, and a cause of chronic childhood constipation and anal fissures (which reversed in 100 percent of cases after all dairy products were discontinued in one study published in the *New England Journal of Medicine*), plus the fact that most people of color cannot digest it (lactose intolerance), you'd think that it would be taken off the menu. Evidenced by lactose intolerance, a common condition, we are not meant to drink mammals' milk after weaning—from any species. With chronic constipation and anal fissures, many children spend the day with belly aches, diarrhea, or constipation, which makes it impossible for them to focus, learn, or enjoy themselves."

These are the challenges CHSF is faced with every day in their fight to bring healthier, plant-based options to schools everywhere.

So, what real-life stories showcase the challenges faced by vegan kids, and what does Amie Hamlin think the future holds in terms of vegan food options?

"Most schools already have a vegan option—peanut butter and jelly," Hamlin says, echoing Dr. Barnard. "And more and more schools *are* offering vegan options! Three public schools in New York City have vegetarian menus, thanks to the work of CHSF, and those menus are vegan half the time. Our recipes have been distributed to 25,000 schools nationwide, including all public schools in California."

All public schools in the third largest state in the United States now have access to vegan recipes for their school's menus. That's 6,299,451 K-12 students who have access to vegan recipe options for lunch they may not even be aware of.

"Most school food service directors want to offer food that kids will eat," Amie says. "So, putting food on the menu is not enough. In fact, doing that without an educational marketing effort in place is a recipe for disaster. It's really important to make eating vegan food cool, and then have the kids/parents/teachers asking for it. It helps if all adults are on board: parents, teachers, administrators, and especially the food service personnel. Without the adults on board, you cannot expect success. With middle and high school, kids can lead the effort to increase these offerings. But they still need to make it desirable among their peers.

"Presentations for how food service directors can make food appealing—with the message of 'take this—it's great'—are important. If the food service people put eight cheeseburgers and two veggie burgers out, what is the message? It's that they expect kids to take the cheeseburgers and not the veggie burger. They should put the veggie burgers first, and put out at least equal numbers. Their language matters a lot, too. I'll never forget: many years ago, there was a food service worker who talked kids out of it, saying, 'Are you sure you want that? It's a veggie burger.' This was in the early nineties, before I even had this job. If they say instead, 'Today, we have the most delicious veggie burgers; you should try them,' it would make a difference."

Can a parent expect to get more vegan options in their schools, from daycare to elementary to high school? Yes. And they can start by contacting CHSF and asking for Amie.

It's up to you, the parent, to make these changes happen.

Which is exactly what we did at our toddlers' daycare when we realized that our monthly tuition for two was going toward the snacks our own kids couldn't enjoy. Aside from fruit, the cart that was wheeled from room to room each day was weighted down with dairy milk and nonvegan snacks. We knew we had to do something to make the situation equitable, so we started with a letter to the corporate office.

Dear XX,

My wife and I have been trying, unsuccessfully, to receive equal treatment at the daycare at Cornell University (Ithaca, NY). For almost three years, we have struggled to understand why we have to provide our own snacks to our TWO children (read = $2,900/month) when other parents don't have to.

We have been told that it's a "budget issue" by the Nutritionist at Cornell, which, of course, is completely untrue since the Center can simply purchase the snacks and beverages required for our children (and others with similar dietary confusions) out of the same budget they are using for the current snacks.

What is it going to take to have nondairy milk, egg-free/ dairy-free snacks, and gluten-free options?

I am at my wits' end over this. I understand our nearly $3,000/month is meaningless to a center in an affluent community that has a waitlist but would assume you'd want to provide excellent client service to all the parents.

Please reply with a phone call at as soon as you have an acceptable solution.

Respectfully,

Eric C Lindstrom

Purposefully written with a rather stern tone, the letter did get the attention of the daycare administrator. They immediately set up a meeting to discuss the matter with someone from HQ. Citing FDA requirements and other nutritional guidelines they were forced to follow based on post–World War II food pyramids, the daycare put up resistance at first since they claimed they were at risk of violating policy, which could affect the daycare's subsidies. However, after keeping on them for another few weeks and asking every day at drop off and pick up, we actually got them to agree to purchase nondairy milk for each room, as well as offer vegan snacks for the kids (while this effort was started for our own vegan kids, it also ended helping out the parents of lactose-intolerant kids).

The daycare has also started a vegetable garden. Abundant with regional bounty, this quarter-acre patch of land teaches young children about where their *food* actually comes from. During the harvest season, this garden is filled with up to twenty little gardeners picking fresh fruit and vegetables and popping some in their mouths along the way.

It dawned on me one day when I was picking the kids up, as they were both crunching on cucumbers, that the daycare hadn't started a slaughterhouse.

Since animals are not food.

I tell my vegan friends and parent of little ones this, and press on, "So then, now tell me why can't everyone be vegan?"

"Because a lot of people enjoy meat," they'll reply.

"A lot of animals enjoy life," I say. I'm done here.

The other day, I was at our kids' daycare, and I took a seat at a tiny table in the center's "pretend" kitchen. In the middle of the table, scattered among plastic fruits and vegetables, was a fake molded roasted chicken. It seemed an odd choice for kids to play with, but I have to remember that others don't see the world through the same lens I do. A friend's three-year-old daughter sat next to me.

She was pouring me pretend tea, being all sweet and innocent.

I picked up the bakelite bird.

"Do you know what this is?" I asked her, pointing at the plastic chicken, knowing I was finally communicating to someone at the same intellectual level as myself and might therefore engage in some spirited dialogue.

"It's a dead bird," I went on, not once thinking about how I could potentially scar her for life while promoting the vegan message.

Without missing a beat, she replied, "No. It's a chicken."

Indoctrination starts early.

Change *can* happen. In fact, students in New York City have recently been treated to new plant-based dishes because of the effort and support by Brooklyn Borough President Eric L. Adams, who happens to be vegan.

Since October 2017, all 1,200 schools in the New York City public school district have been offering at least one vegan entrée. Read that sentence again. If New York City can do it, then certainly your small school in rural Illinois can, too.

Previously, New York City students already had vegan options that consisted of fruits, vegetables, and peanut butter and jelly sandwiches. These lucky students will now be able to choose from such creative vegan options as Mexicali Chili, Lentil Stew, Lentil Sloppy Joes, Braised Black Beans with Plantains, and Zesty BBQ Crunchy Tofu. This move not only shows support for kids who may want to eat vegan and support healthier food options; it also potentially saves hundreds of animals each year.

And it turns out that it's Amie Hamlin's organization, The Coalition for Healthy School Food (CHSF), which is behind this new initiative. To date, they've worked with the city's department of education to help three New York City schools—Active Learning Elementary School in Queens (PS244), Peck Slip School in Manhattan (PS343), and The Bergen Elementary School (PS1) in Brooklyn—to transition to an all-vegetarian menu. PS1 Principal Arlene Ramos revealed that students asked for healthier, meatless options and that she is excited to be able to introduce the new menu. Brooklyn Borough President Adams—who adopted a vegan diet in 2016 to conquer his type 2 diabetes—also supports the menu update. "It is particularly exciting to learn that this is a youth-driven initiative," Adams tells me. "Our children understand that a healthy meal is the best fuel for a quality education, and I am pleased to work with CHSF as we advance a wholesome whole-food vision for our youngest Brooklynites and their families."

Earlier this year, seven schools within the Los Angeles School District also launched a vegan lunch pilot program, to which students have, thus far, responded with glowing reviews.

As the saying goes, "Good things come to people who wait, but better things come to those who go out and get them."

You've given birth to your vegan baby and nurtured them with all the fruits and vegetables and whole grains you could. You've cried watching your vegan toddler step onto the kindergarten school bus for the first time and packed healthy vegan lunches throughout elementary school. You tried to help your vegan middle schooler with their math homework (all while not understanding any of it). You helped to guide them through the challenges of high school, and then you helped to unpack your twenty-year-old's Honda at college. What happens now?

The Ethical Choices Program (ECP) is a not-for-profit that reaches high school and college students. According to their website, they are "dedicated to inspiring this generation to realize the importance and responsibility of being informed and to understand the power and influence they wield to make the world a better place through food choices."

Their website continues: "We focus our education program efforts on high school and college students, an age group that is more open and willing to examine our cultural choices than any other. And rather than telling those students what to think or feel, ECP educators help students find answers for themselves. We encourage students to think about their own experiences and examine their choices anew through an informed lens. Through respectful, non-judgmental and open dialogue students are encouraged to choose a path that accords with their own values and beliefs."

Lorena Mucke, the founder and chief executive officer of ECP, is the heart and soul of the organization who has been leading it since it was founded in late 2015. Her vision for a nonprofit education program that informs teenagers and adults about the effects of food choices on our health, the environment, and animals has been realized, and she continues to reach students and others throughout the United States, Canada, and Australia.

Lorena has an undergraduate degree in zoology from Texas A&M University and a graduate degree in ecology and sustainable development from Instituto Universitario Patricios in Argentina. Since her teen years, she has been an advocate for the environment and has lectured extensively on related topics in the United States, Argentina, and Bolivia. She began ECP by personally lecturing to students in the greater Atlanta area, which she continues to do regularly. Her own vegan kids inspired her to start the program. Lorena says:

As a mother raising three vegan children (a sixteen-year-old boy and nine-year-old twin girls) and an educator for the last twelve years who encourages teens to critically think about their food choices and how they impact their own health and the world around them, I've learned much about how children and teens (and their parents!) view food and the animals we call food," Lorena says. "Children and teens are naturally compassionate, but society has taught them to view farm animals as commodities.

When these students become aware that farm animals are no different than the animals they call 'pets,' they begin to make the connection. Scientifically speaking, farm animals are able to feel pain, interact with other animals and humans, form bonds, play, and enjoy exercising their nature-given instincts. Through ECP, students come to understand what these animals endure in farms and slaughterhouses, and they feel somewhat betrayed by society—and their parents. One of the most common questions we've heard is, 'How come we didn't know?' The beauty is that teens are ready to change the world, once given new information. Instead of accepting the status quo, they are eager to step up to the challenge if we only give them the chance.

Children and teens are also naturally inquisitive. They appreciate when we are forthcoming and when we offer factual information. After all, they can fact-check what we say in a few seconds on their phones. They truly embrace the phrase 'information is power.' However, teens over the years have shared with me that they feel underestimated, which I think is one of the biggest mistakes we make as adults when we relate to them. We must recognize that teens are the future decision-makers and game-changers. Most importantly, we must act accordingly.

Teens don't like to be told what to eat or not to eat. Nobody does. That's why one of the most fulfilling aspects about my job as an educator is to expose teens to age-appropriate information, to which they might have never been exposed, and allow them to ask questions and assimilate the new information. Most important, we provide them with tools so they feel empowered to make changes if they so desire. In turn, these teens share with their parents and peers the new information and make different choices if they want to and when they can—by cooking something at home, choosing anew what to eat at the school cafeteria or when they go out to eat with friends, etc.

Teenagers are more aware than we realize about the urgent health and environmental problems we are facing and the tremendous cruelty animals are subjected to. What they need are adults who are willing to discuss these issues in a frank and factual manner; who offer them to be part of the solution; who recognize that teens' real fears of being stuck in a food system benefits no one; who are willing to learn and to be open-minded to new information; who support their choices as long as they promote their well-being and make the world a better place; and who are willing to be the change they want to see in the world.

Flash forward a full decade from this moment. Your little eight-year-old vegan has become a bright-eyed, optimistic young vegan adult, navigating their life through a four-year college or university. Like Ben.

"For me, being vegan is about reconciling my knowledge of climate change with my actions," says Ben, a twenty-year-old junior and government major at Cornell University. "Specifically, it's about reconciling that knowledge with my personal agency and my individual conscience.

"Once you have learned about the cause and effects of climate change, you cannot unlearn. Once you are aware of the human suffering that climate change causes and will cause, you can ignore your own complicity—but never un-know—and attempt to carry on with business as usual (this is relatively easy as a middle-class American college student). Or, you can try to change your behavior in a way that reduces your contribution to the climate holocaust and provides your conscience with some relief.

"As human beings, our actions or inactions have power and the ability to influence climate change. We have agency. By being vegan, I decrease the demand for animal products and withhold financial support from the meat and dairy industry, while increasing demand and lending financial support to sources of food that have a much smaller impact on the environment. Additionally, I increase the visibility of veganism and may even convert a few "woke" friends.

"Veganism for me is also a more individual matter of conscience. Regardless of the magnitude my actions have on the meat industry or climate change, I am still confronted with my complicity in ocean acidification, drought, human displacement, natural disasters, etc., that disproportionately affect marginalized populations and will affect all of human civilization in the near future. Being vegan is a way for me to reduce my complicity in climate change for my own sake, so that I can better live with myself. It is a personal matter of principle and integrity and a way to reconcile my knowledge, values, means, and actions as best I can."

Ben is part of what has been referred to as Generation Z. This generation is embracing a food trend that replaces animal products with plant-based alternatives—and this generation is set to save the planet. Startups that make fake meat and seafood are targeting college and university cafeterias for distribution because it's where they expect to find enthusiastic consumers. This was the case with vegan mayo manufacturer Hampton Creek, which, in one fell swoop, replaced egg-based mayo on all Ivy League campuses in 2016 with the healthier plant-based Just Mayo.

And no one even noticed.

Generation Z includes people born between the mid-1990s and mid-2000s, which means the oldest members of the demographic are currently getting ready to graduate college. This group makes up a quarter of the United States population and will account for 40 percent of all consumers by 2020—and they are embracing veganism. Generation Z, according to *Business Insider*, is responsible for the success of the alt-meat market: "The substitute meat market is expected to grow 8.4% annually over the next three years, reaching $5.2 billion globally by 2020." Ben is part of an elite group of young people about to embark on "real life," and they are making a difference for future generations by choosing to go vegan.

Ben's best friend at Cornell is Sarvar, a computer science major and one of at least five students I know personally who have chosen to go vegan.

"I grew up in an immigrant family that held onto its culture through food," Sarvar says. "Everything I ate, from palak paneer to butter chicken to yogurt, was inextricable from centuries of a cultural history my parents had inherited and wanted to pass on to me. Food was one of the ways love manifested in my family (like many families)—I could smell the naan and butter from my mother's kitchen as soon as I reached my street, and even before I stepped inside I could feel her embrace and hear my dad's laughter."

Sarvar's family moved to the United States and New York City from India in 2005 when Sarvar was five. While his vegan journey began outside the house, Saryar's parents remain an important part of his life.

"I love my parents," Sarvar confesses. "I am unbelievably lucky in that I can say I come from a stable family that has always provided for me and made me feel accepted. It is because I love my parents that I now hesitate before picking up a piece of naan slathered in butter and turn away from chicken altogether. Love should be built on foundations of trust and care and certainly not constructed within a framework of exploitation."

While meat consumption in India is relatively low, their 75 million dairy farms now produce more milk than all of the European Union. India remains the largest producer of milk and milk products in the world. Milk is in most recipes and on most menus, and based on the 1.43 billion population of India, their enormous animal agriculture industry is obviously a major contributor to global warming, ranking them fourth in the world.

Sarvar is aware of his own impact on the planet and believes that, by going vegan, he can make a difference for his entire family.

"It is because I love my parents that I've chosen to go vegan. We're pumping greenhouse gases into our atmosphere at ever-increasing rates, and that is the greatest threat to love I can imagine," Sarvar says. "I could continue to eat dairy products and meat and buy leather wallets, and my life (for the next few decades, at least) would be largely unaffected by the majority of issues associated with climate change. But my greatest fear, as cliché as it may be, is lying on my deathbed, surrounded by my own children, knowing I did not give them a world as full of opportunity as mine. I know it sounds dire, and I know it's unbelievably easy to distance oneself from such a grim future, but if we maintain our status quo, this world won't exist in the same way it does now. And we almost definitely won't exist in the same way we do now, if at all.

"I have had all of the privileges of a healthy earth, and to increasingly strip future generations of those same privileges seems analogous to murder."

Sarvar is part of a handful of Cornell students whom I am fortunate enough to interact with regularly and provide support and guidance to as they navigate veganism. Some of these students approached veganism from the animal rights perspective, having watched the 2005 documentary *Earthlings*, and some were thinking about their health, but most are concerned about the environment.

"I did initially embrace veganism for the environmental benefits, but I have also grown to value the choice for its implications on animal welfare," Sarvar says. "Food packed with the milk from a tortured mother is not a meal of love, regardless of my mother's intentions or ignorance in its creation. I've come to view it as wearing blood diamonds around your neck—it may look good or taste good, but somewhere deep down, I'll always know the kind of pain that my own preference demanded."

What would Sarvar say to parents who are thinking about raising their kids vegan?

"I'm really not here to convince you to go vegan or to tell you it's easy—it's not. There are mornings when I wake up fighting that eternal internal battle over cream cheese, and it takes everything I have to grab the box of Tofutti over the Philadelphia. Every day, though, it gets a little easier. I've started to imagine the wrinkles around my father's eyes when he makes some cheesy joke or the benevolence in my mother's laughter after hearing it. And here's the thing: somewhere along the line, the Tofutti starts tasting better. It's guilt-free, it's wholesome food, it is love embodied."

Because of my wife Jen's work, I've been very fortunate to have lived on Cornell University campus for a number of years and have been able to both interact with these two-thousand-plus Ivy League students and gauge the vegan climate in higher ed. Turns out, dining halls nationwide are embracing veganism and making plant-based foods an emphasis on their menus. In fact, most dining rooms clearly label all dietary preferences, and some will take recommendations from students and/or prepare special meals depending on students' dietary preferences.

There is everything at Cornell, from a tofu scramble bar with tater tots to Meatless Monday options that look and taste like real meat (in fact, I often wonder if the students know they're not eating animal protein as they pile it on their plate). In the years we've lived at Cornell, we've seen a major shift toward more and more creative vegan food options and events. In fact, Cornell University scored a 91 percent satisfaction rating in a poll conducted by PETA for student satisfaction for vegan options.

Meanwhile, in nearby New Haven, Connecticut, vegan protein innovator Beyond Meat announced in the fall of 2017 that their Beyond Burger will be offered at all thirteen on-campus dining halls at Yale. This 315-year-old Ivy League institution is widely recognized as a thought leader in hospitality and dining innovation, so for it to be the first ever university to carry this amazing burger is setting the bar for other universities and college campuses to follow. As more dining halls on campuses begin offering these vegan options, the popularity will only increase. The market is there with the greatest generation of students embracing veganism.

It's easier than ever to be vegan.

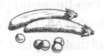

13
HARAMBE: A GORILLA DIES IN CINCINNATI

"Animals are not products. Life doesn't have a price."
—*Anonymous*

Back in May 2016, a rambunctious three-year-old boy fell into a lowland gorilla enclosure at the Cincinnati Zoo and Botanical Garden. What unfolded, for the most part, was caught on amateur cellphone video. Harambe, a seventeen-year-old 440-pound gorilla proceeded to fetch the small child from the water feature in his cell and seemed to enjoy poking, prodding, and tossing the little boy around, obviously terrifying his parents and everyone watching.

Apparently, the spirited boy climbed a three-foot-tall fence, crawled through four feet of bushes, and then fell fifteen feet into a moat of shallow water close to where Harambe was sitting. Some people criticized the parents of the little boy, but I can tell you that our son Cooper would have done the same thing. There are just some kids who cannot be contained.

Of course, the zoo responded with bloodshed. The authorities felt they had no choice but to kill Harambe with a single gunshot—sniper-style from above the enclosure. This seventeen-year-old gorilla who never knew freedom, whose already stressful space was disrupted by a surprise visit from a small child, was killed in broad daylight. Killing Harambe seemed to be the only logical choice to make in order to save the boy's life.

But *was* it really?

Video evidence shows the boy wasn't actually (intentionally) being hurt by the gorilla. In fact, Harambe seemed to be helping by pulling him out of the water. What *would* have happened if they had left the gorilla alone with the boy longer? Would he have lost interest and let the boy go? Would the gorilla have ended up cuddling or nurturing his newfound friend? What if the zoo had coaxed Harambe away from the boy with his usual feeding routine? Or, what if the gorilla himself willingly handled the boy over?

So many unanswered questions. We'll never know, because the authorities felt they couldn't take any of these unknown risks, preferring to kill him.

Conclusion: a human boy's life was considered more valuable than that of a gorilla's. This leads us to question: why was the boy's life considered more valuable than the gorilla's? Are human lives more important than other animals'?

Had literally any other species of animal fallen into that enclosure instead, the zoo most likely would have stayed back and let nature take its course. This idea that the boy's life was more valuable than the gorilla's brings to the forefront, once again, this idea of *speciesism*, which we examined in chapter three. One species is considered more important than another. Pigs, who are more intelligent than dogs, are bred and butchered for meat while the family dog looks on and feeds from the table scraps.

Here is another description of speciesism:

speciesism [ˈspēSHēˌzizəm, spēsē-/]
[noun] the assumption of human superiority leading to the exploitation of animals

At what point, if ever, will we look the other way in regard to speciesism? Will veganism become so accepted that the majority population will eventually make the connection and realize this is a planet shared by all?

If we believe a human's life is more important than a gorilla's, then is a *frog's* life as important as a gorilla's?

In Ithaca where we live, we are surrounded by colleges and universities, lakes and wineries, and bucolic rolling hills. However, we have very little to do with the little ones on weekends, which is why we go to the Sciencenter. I bring our two budding scientists to the hands-on science museum pretty much once a week. They have science displays, an outdoor playground, and cool experiments and activities to keep our toddlers occupied for hours on end.

And they also have frogs.

And snakes and fish and horseshoe crabs and a variety of other small amphibians and marine life, all held captive in cages, glass tanks, and terrariums in one small room within the 18,000-square foot museum.

When Harambe was killed, I voiced my opinion, which is actually an undisputed fact, that gorillas don't belong in Cincinnati in the first place. Penguins don't belong in Pittsburgh. And giraffes don't belong in Jacksonville. They just don't.

I mention this fact, and a friend, who likes to poke at our vegan lifestyle, took time to comment and start a "discussion."

"So, you're saying zoos are bad?" he asked, knowing full well what my answer was going to be. Nonvegans do this all the time.

"Yes. There really is no such thing as a 'good zoo' or a 'good aquarium.' Animals don't deserve to be imprisoned for human entertainment."

"You think Harambe would have been better off in the wild?"

"Of course. It's where he belongs."

"And you won't take your kids to zoos or aquariums as part of your 'vegan agenda'?"

"No. They can learn all they need to learn from books and the internet. As it is, Cooper knows more about dinosaurs than any other animal, and, not surprisingly, he's never actually *seen* one before. We won't support them."

"But, you take your kids to the Sciencenter."

Long silence.

Caught. Off guard.

Of course, the answer was "yes" and "often," and I knew where his line of questioning was heading. If we were "true vegans," we wouldn't support even a small hands-on science museum in our small town because they feature smaller, mostly local, animals in their glass-lined prisons. I had no response. I had to dig deeper to truly wrap my mind around his point. Sure, I can use the opportunity to educate my kids on the fact that these animals belong in the wild and that, to us, the life of a frog is as important as the life of a gorilla, a snake, a lizard, and a fish. No matter the size or species of an animal, they should be allowed their freedom.

Yet, there I am. Supporting their imprisonment. To this day, I still think about it every time we go back to the Sciencenter.

What *is* the value of an unborn chick versus an adult chicken, especially in classrooms where the practice of hatching is meant to educate?

Cindy Ford, a vegan parent of two, is a home cook who enjoys writing about all things vegan. She lives in Columbus just an hour and a half from where Harambe spent his last days of his imprisoned life, and she's also the HappyCow vegan ambassador for the city. Active in her daughters' lives, she became a Parent Teacher Organization (PTO) activist when her girls came home with the flyer saying they would be hatching eggs in their classroom.

Okay, vegans, what's wrong with hatching eggs in the classroom?

"I think this is an important question," says Cindy. "Raising chicks in the classroom may seem like an innocuous educational lesson, but it's important to ask questions to uncover the real issues involved. The answers will shed light to the very nature of the problems, and there are many. When I dealt with this issue, the first question I asked my daughter's teacher was, 'Where were these chicks obtained?' The follow-up question was (and I asked this of all the teachers in my daughter's grade), 'What will happen to the chicks after the project?' While these seem like simple questions, they were never asked before. They had never been thought of much by the parents before me. The only concern by (nonvegan) friends was whether or not they would be one of the 'lucky' families to bring home the chicks post-lesson (my suburban town outside of Columbus allows backyard hens)."

Cindy educated the educators and shed light on the downside of hatching in the classroom, while also outing herself as a "crazy vegan."

"I truly think that becoming vegan has changed me in every sense," she says. "It has made me more thoughtful and aware of the animals that are around us. I continually wonder what is happening to them in relationship to humans. Is it positive or negative? Unfortunately, I've realized that very few animals have benefited from human contact.

"At our elementary school, the fertilized chicken eggs were mailed via the post office to the school from a hatchery. I had no idea that this was common practice. After hatching, our school allowed the chicks to go home with parental permission. While hens are allowed in my city, roosters are not. In my community, hens are permitted so that my neighbors can exploit them for their eggs.

"Unfortunately, all unwanted chicks are sent to the local university's extension program (Ohio State University). OSU has been responsible for giving the unwanted animals to local farmers. I was informed by the extension liaison that the animals would likely be used for laying purposes and possibly meat. As she explained, they are 'meat animals.'"

Meat animals. From an in-classroom science experiment to the dinner table. These adorable chirping chicks grow up before the kids' eyes, only to later become a McNugget. Could you imagine, right after these chicks were hatched, if the teacher asked, "Who wants to eat one first?"

That's what's going on here.

"Despite the certain fate of these animals, I think an (un)expected issue with raising chicks in the classroom is the emotional attachment that the children develop by raising and caring for them," Cindy continues. "This was definitely an issue that our family dealt with. My daughter quickly became attached to one chick in particular. She named him Brownie, and he was adopted by a family who had the intention of eating the bird. My family was really concerned and wanted nothing more than to save my daughter's favorite chick. In the end, I was able to rescue him and four other chicks from the project by finding them refuge at the local animal sanctuary. Guess what? The other children in the class also wanted the chicks to live (even though most were eating chicken regularly)."

The 2012 documentary *Peaceable Kingdom* uncovers more about the connections kids make to animals and how their upbringing and education leads them down certain paths. The film explores the awakening conscience of several people who grew up in traditional farming culture and who have now come to question the basic assumptions of their way of life. One person featured is Harold Brown, who happens to work at my local co-op in Ithaca and who has become an outspoken animal rights activist.

Harold was raised on a dairy farm in south central Michigan and spent much of his childhood raising cows as part of his 4-H youth program. Through Harold's own accounts, and emotional footage of other young people in the same program, it becomes evident fairly quickly in the film that the kids form strong, emotional bonds with the animals they are raising as they compete for "Best in Show," only to find out that the cows are later sold for auction and either live out the rest of their lives in a constant state of pregnancy/lactation or are slaughtered for meat.

The World Dairy Expo, held in Madison, Wisconsin, is the world's largest dairy expo. This is where cows go to have their udders lotioned up so they can be judged in the arena not unlike a beauty pageant; except, of course, that there is nothing beautiful about the event. These animals lead a life of servitude, are forced to give up their offspring, and travel for sometimes hundreds of miles in a hot trailer, only to be judged on how laden they can become with milk—sometimes so much so that they can't walk normally. These innocent cows were born and bred to be impregnated, milked, shown off, auctioned off, and murdered.

Imagine raising a show dog who wins a blue ribbon at Westminster, only to be forced to auction off your dog—and later you discover she was killed for meat. (For the record, adopt/don't shop; please find your companion animal at a rescue.)

A dog is a cow is a cat is a pig is a human.

Harold eventually realized that all animals, including humans, exist for their own reasons and with their own interests. He is now a strong voice for animal rights, and he has started a website called FarmKind.org, which intends to be a resource for farmers who want to make the transition from animal-based to plant-based agriculture. It also teaches consumers a different perspective on how food is produced and helps those who desire to reconnect with the land and become farmers to support local food production, environmental and social justice issues, and the rights of all living beings to be cohabitants of this planet in order to create a more peaceful world.

It's a known fact that children, like Harold when he was younger, form bonding relationships with animals. I read somewhere that when asked to name the ten most important individuals in their lives, seven- to ten-year-olds on average included two pets. Many children (and adults) consider their pets as family members, and some children consider their pets as though they were younger siblings, peers, or even as security-providing attachment figures. Even children who know that the farm animals they help raise will one day potentially become their dinner still form relationships that are not unlike those with their pets. Why are some animals arbitrarily considered family members and not others?

The human-animal bond is a mutually beneficial and dynamic relationship that positively influences the health and well-being of both parties. While many of us understand the benefits of positive interactions with animals in our lives, an emerging body of research is recognizing the impact the human-animal bond can have on individual and community health. The bond is even more evident within each species as most animals form a bond with their offspring at birth. Mothers are what keeps the planet alive.

"I think a part of the issue that a lot of people don't consider when it comes to chick rearing is the strong maternal instincts of hens," says Cindy. "Like humans, mother hens spend time with their young teaching them life skills. Hens are also known for being extremely protective of their babies. So, with a class raising these birds from an incubator, they are essentially destroying the maternal bond between a mother and her young. This class (along with all of the classes before them) is a part of a system that creates orphans and then essentially throws away the ones that aren't deemed valuable.

"When schools teach children to be kind and respect animals (by teaching them how to care for them during the time they are in the classroom), they are being inconsistent. In essence, a chick-hatching lesson continues to teach children that animals are disposable and can be used and discarded like objects. This is a contradiction."

What happens after the lesson is completed and the chicks are ready to be disposed?

"It potentially creates a burden to families," Cindy says. "My family was not the first family in our school to look for a safe place for the chicks to live out the remainder of their lives. The question becomes, 'Where can I take them?' For me, I was quite lucky. I had been really involved at the time with our local animal sanctuary, Sunrise Sanctuary in Marysville, Ohio.

"While they were at or near capacity, as many sanctuaries are, they were willing to take five roosters from the chick-hatching program. Being at capacity is such a common thread among sanctuaries, and programs such as these only exacerbate the situation."

Tamerlaine Farm Sanctuary, in Montague Township, New Jersey, urges schools to not participate in this type of school project. They made a deal with a teacher who reached out to them to ask about stopping the program in their school. In return, the sanctuary agreed to give the kids a presentation and educate them about the animals at their sanctuary and what they can do to help animals. If a sanctuary is located nearby any schools with such programs, a field trip instead of a hatching project is the best way to interact with animals, offering a memorable learning experience.

Finally, there are also concerns about human and animal health within these in-classroom hatching programs.

"An aspect that a school needs to be concerned with in terms of bringing live animals into a school is the associated health risk. The Center for Disease Control (CDC) updates their site annually, providing information on the number of infections due to the handling of live chickens. They also give information on ways to reduce salmonella infections due to contact with backyard chickens. The information includes people who are most susceptible to disease. That would include young children (under the age of five—kindergarteners). More recently, the CDC has been urging people to *quit hugging their chickens!*"

With as many as 375 known cases per year and over seventy hospitalizations, these programs are putting thousands of school-age kids at risk. What can you do if this is happening near you? Well, what did Cindy do?

"The first thing I did was reach out to my daughter's teachers via email, gathering information. It didn't get me very far. One of my daughter's teachers responded that he appreciated my 'pro-animal-life' views (his words, not mine) but that, for many children, this lesson would be the first time some children would get to deal with live animals.

"It's interesting how we equate value in terms of subjugating animals, isn't it? Lessons like these teach children to turn living beings into objects. Their own life (the chicks) only have value in relation to how humans can use them, and if we can't use them (or we are finished with them) then they can be forgotten and discarded.

"After not getting very far with my daughter's teacher, I moved onto our school's Parent Teacher Organization (PTO). At the time, I was a co-vice-president. I had learned that it's easier to change things from within, and getting involved with the PTO was a way to get more involved with the school. At one of our meetings, I put the chick-rearing issue on our agenda. I addressed the parents, teachers, and principal, and that was *not* easy. While I knew I was trying to do something positive, I was doing it alone. One member of the PTO board said, 'You really like to save chickens, I really like to eat them.'"

Cognitive dissonance strikes again.

Cognitive dissonance [cog·ni·tive dis·so·nance]
[noun] the state of having inconsistent thoughts, beliefs, or attitudes,
especially as relating to behavioral decisions and attitude change

You know it's not right and you know in your heart it's not what you believe—but you do it anyway. You support big agriculture and big dairy even though you know it's wrong—you separate what is truth from what you want to believe. Another example might be the guilt someone feels when eating a Cinnaholic vegan gourmet cinnamon roll while on a diet. They know they shouldn't be eating it, but they like sweets. Two values—health and sweets—in conflict, creating a feeling of guilt.

Yet another example might be when people who enjoy eating meat are presented with imagery, or facts, about the known cruelty and *obvious* suffering of animals that colludes with their innate sense of compassion. This is a conflicting set of values—eating meat and being compassionate—these emotions cannot coexist in one person.

No matter what anyone tells you, you cannot truly be an animal lover and not be vegan. Cognitive dissonance happens every day in society. This is not a matter of opinion. It simply is not right. Cindy's quest continued.

"There were other board members who were supportive of my initiative, but no one was really my ally. I presented my case, which included the compassionate argument behind ending the hatching program (the children's attachment and then rescuing some of the chicks), and I also presented the health issue. I personally think that the health issue is the most valuable argument in a school setting. While many people pick and choose the animals that they feel compassionate towards, people care very deeply about the safety of their children. So, I showed the health risks associated with the lesson by bringing in information from the CDC. I spoke about CDC recommendations, the health risk, and also about the school's liability if a child got sick from a zoonotic disease.

"Unfortunately, at this time the school is continuing the lesson. They have shortened the length of time that the animals are in the classroom to half of the time it was, and they no longer allow families to take the animals home. Maybe they think they have solved the issue of having chicks in the classroom as children are not getting as attached and there is less exposure to possible disease. I'm not sure.

"I think I would've been much more successful with this issue if I had parental allies within my children's school. One parent may not be enough to fight a system of exploitation within an elementary school or a school district. However, a school is an extension of the families in the community, so it may take many more voices to get heard. However, I think that I put a crack into the system, and it is only time before this all falls."

Cindy's activism for her beliefs and for her daughters extends past the classroom, too. When asked about allowing her daughters to attend field trips to zoos, she feels just as strongly about the message that is being conveyed to young minds. As a general rule, vegans avoid zoos, marine aquariums, and circuses—essentially anywhere animals are caged, confined, abused, or used as objects for entertainment.

"Every family is different. What unites vegan families is addressing nonvegan issues such as field trips (and chick hatching) within schools," says Cindy. "There are definitely times when I have considered home-schooling because I see so many issues with the inconsistencies being taught in regards to loving animals and being a part of their exploitation. However, I realize that while my husband and I can teach our children our values, it is how we handle undesirable situations, as vegan parents, that show our children what it means to live vegan. I use the failings in school as teachable lessons for my children. If we take our children out of school and raise them within a vegan bubble, will they know what to do when faced with challenges? I think that we can be great advocates for animals and children at the same time by having them in public/private school.

"Almost every year, there is a questionable field trip for both my children. The trips are either to the local zoo or an 'ole timey' farm run by our state park department. My initial instinct is to just pull them from the trip and keep them home. If the trips occur during the spring, there is usually a screening of an animal documentary to take them to (which I find to be more educational than the zoo!). But more recently, I have started to give my children the option of going.

"That may seem very nonvegan, right? But here's why I think it can be valuable lesson for them. If my child decides to go (or not go), they are making the choice. They are taking responsibility for missing the fieldtrip and the consequence of it. That consequence includes missing time with their friends from their class, and possibly being on the outside of a shared class experience. However, if my children choose to go, they realize that they will be there to 'bear witness,' much like those before them, such as activists Joanne McArthur or Shaun Monson of *We Animals* and *Earthlings*, respectively. They have documented animals in the worst conditions and extreme cruelty at the hand of humans. My children, if they choose to go, will be expected to recognize what it means to be a captive, an animal whose life was stolen from them to be used as a prop in our world.

"As a vegan parent, we strive to impart a compassionate perspective in our children; therefore, we must trust that they, because of the knowledge and values we have imparted, will make sense of the trip in their own way, a way that is likely markedly different from their classmates.

"In terms of addressing the issue of a missed field trip with a teacher, this can be touchy. Most kids love these field trips, and it's extremely uncommon for a child to miss them, which can make it a difficult and/or an uncomfortable topic to discuss with a teacher. Over the years, however, I have found that emailing the teacher is the best way to communicate the issue. This communication allows the parent to carefully express the family's core values and why the field trip goes against those values. Pro tip: be as polite and nonjudgmental as possible. This can be hard, but most of us were not born vegan. Being understanding and nonjudgmental may just open the teacher's eyes just a little."

Parenting vegan kids is a lot of work, but does all this effort go unnoticed?

"While my vegan friends have appreciated my efforts in speaking up at the elementary school, I have never been thanked by other parents in regards to my stance on chick rearing or field trips.

"However, our PTO was thanked for offering a nondairy option at its annual Ice Cream Social. I had everything to do with getting that on the menu, but I let the PTO take the credit. The parent who thanked us had a child with a dairy allergy, and allergies are socially acceptable. In comparison, being consistent in morals and actions (being vegan) is not as acceptable or recognized and not a social norm. Behind my back, I heard that I'm called 'that vegan mom,' but I wear that as a badge.

I'm really proud to be vegan, and everything that it means to be vegan. I seek to do good in this world. I want to be kind to others, be it human or animal."

If children don't have access to farm sanctuaries, how would you go about introducing them to live animals?

"I'm starting to realize that there are sanctuaries all over the place!" Cindy exclaims. "While we have one that's about forty-five minutes away, we will occasionally make a trip to a different sanctuary as part of our family road trips. I've been to a few now, and I realize just how different each one is! They are special places. If you can make a trip to one, it can change you. I remember the first time that I met a steer as a vegan. I almost cried. I told him that I was sorry over and over. I felt bad, and I still feel bad for the things that we (humans) do to animals.

"However, if going to a sanctuary is not something a family can do, there are other ways to introduce children to live animals. There are animal documentaries that are shown at the movie theatre. While my children choose not go to the zoo, they still get to enjoy wild animals on the movie screen. Both of my daughters have loved our 'field trips' to the movies. There are also documentaries on Netflix and at the library. While at the library, there are also plenty of books to check out. I find these options so much more educational than a school trip to the zoo!

"Personally, I'd love to save the money to take our children on some trips to see animals in the wild. On my bucket list is a trip to Costa Rica to see sloths." (Sloths happen to be Cindy's spirit animal.)

Going back to the basics, does Cindy agree that kids are born compassionate?

"Of course! As children, we are born both curious *and* compassionate," Cindy says. "Compassion is a part of humanity, and this is why there is a vegan movement. We have to be conditioned starting from childhood to compartmentalize our love for certain animals. Hence, showing compassion toward some animals and not others.

"An interesting story of compassion relates back to the chick rescue. As I mentioned, my daughter's classmate had adopted several of the chicks from the classroom project. Her family had every intention of exploiting those animals for their eggs. If any of those chicks were male, they had planned on eating them. Any hens in their flock who stopped laying would be eaten, also. Their family had no issue with this, and these were the values they were passing on to their children. These parents had informed me that their child knew the difference between "food animals" and pets. However, after I convinced the parents to release the chicks to me, their child asked their father if we could rescue *all* of the chicks.

"Regardless of the parents' attempt to re-program their child into believing that there are 'food animals' and pets, the child chose compassion. Compassion is where our hearts exist naturally.

"If we think deeper about our innate feelings of compassion, it makes sense why people shy away from undercover videos showing any kind of abuse (towards humans and nonhumans). Currently, undercover videos exposing animal abuse are extremely accessible. In fact, a person has to go out of his or her way to *not* watch them. However, I think a good question is, 'Why do people actively seek to *not* learn the truth?' I honestly believe that people don't want to know so they cannot be responsible for making a change in their lives. It is much more convenient to practice avoidance than to change their lives (i.e., going vegan)."

Even though children may come into this world with an instinct to help others, it is our job as parents to nurture and teach them about giving. As we know, so many negative experiences can darken perspectives and turn us off from wanting to help others. However, in order to keep the chain of kindness growing in the world, we need to guide our children to see past those discouraging experiences and to try again, and again, and again.

And again.

14

WHERE TO GO: TRAVELING WITH YOUR LITTLE VEGANS

"There are no foreign lands. It is the traveler only who is foreign."
—*Robert Louis Stevenson*

It's better to see something once than to hear about it a hundred times. Exploring the world with your kids is one of the most rewarding (and exhausting) things you can do as a parent. To be able to fill their brains with real experiences and new locations feeds their hungry little minds.

When we travel, it's oftentimes challenging to find vegan food on the road and in the airports. Since we've become seasoned vegan travelers, we've also learned to pack plenty of snacks before leaving the house.

Our usual checklist: snacks, water, juice boxes (*don't* squeeze them!), fruit and veggie pouches, and a cooler with ice packs. Plus, our portable DVD player if the trip is longer than a few hours. We keep handing back to the hangry kids in the back seat: fruit pouches, bags of chips, apples, orange slices, and the occasional Nugo pretzel bar (seek these out, trust me). This keeps them content for a while, though never as long as we'd like.

The following are a few tips for *your* next vegan travel adventure.

Go online well before you plan to leave and search for "health-food shops" and "vegan restaurants" near where you're staying. Google maps has made this simple. Find your destination on a map and type "vegan" in the search box. Little pins will drop where there are vegan options listed. You can also check with HappyCow.net or download their handy app for finding places to eat along the way.

We've often found that restaurants from different cultures provide more vegan options than your typical mainstream family restaurant. We eat a lot of Korean and Japanese food as well as Mexican. It also makes sense to email or call the hotel or visitors bureau in advance for vegan, and veg-friendly, restaurant suggestions in the area.

On a tight travel budget? Request a hotel room with a mini-fridge or small kitchenette. In fact, since my wife has celiac disease, the hotels are legally required to provide us with a fridge for her "medication," which is usual gluten-free bread and other gluten-free snacks. Stay near a Trader Joe's or Whole Foods if possible or, better yet, a farmer's market. Purchase foods that don't require cooking, such as fruit, fresh veggies with hummus, prepared salads, couscous, and quinoa. To make it more fun, we let our kids pick a new or different-looking food each time we're on vacation (with mixed results).

Bring your favorite carton, or single-serving box, of plant-based milk from home. If you are flying, pack it in your checked suitcase since it won't get through customs on your carry-on for security reasons. We've never encountered a hotel breakfast buffet that didn't allow us to bring our own plant-based milk to the table. Many of these buffets have vegan breakfast cereals and oatmeal, and adding a splash of vanilla almond milk kicks it up a notch. A carton usually lasts our entire trip.

It also helps to bring your own packaged foods, such as granola bars, power bars (Nugo Nutrition are our favorites, did I mention that already?), cookies, fruit bars, crackers, seasoned chickpeas, rice cakes, nuts and seeds in baggies, and even instant oatmeal packets that can be made with hot water in your hotel room. Or, if you're adventurous, you can be like vegan MacGyver and make a vegan grilled cheese sandwich with the hotel's iron.

Don't assume that airlines will have plant-based food options, so be prepared for flights as well. We always pack two sandwiches, pre-cut and in locktop containers, to bring on a plane, and plenty of snacks for all family members. Some airports have more vegan options than others, but it's always good to be ready for delayed flights, especially during the winter months.

Many mainstream restaurants will accommodate vegans, but you have to be clear. If you are in a city where the main language is not English, do your best to translate "no animal products." In our travels, we have encountered dozens of restaurant staff members who have never even heard of a plant-based diet and don't know what "vegan" means. But if you explain nicely that pizza can easily be made without cheese and that pasta can easily be made without butter, they will (usually) happily accommodate you. And, you get to educate people at the same time.

Pro tip: If you tell your server that the kids are *allergic* to dairy and eggs, the kitchen will usually be more responsive, as opposed to trying to accommodate vegans.

When eating out while traveling, we have had good luck at buffets and salad bars because they usually offer many fresh, vegan options for a pay-one-price perk.

Now, let's get real for a minute.

The reason so many parents choose to feed their kids fast food is cost and convenience. Plus, fast food restaurants and fast casual franchises are somewhat obligated to put up with kids. Luckily, there are vegan options at many fast food restaurants now, so you can still hit the drive-thru on the way home from ballet.

Here is an easy-to-use guide on how to order vegan at some of the top fast food restaurants in the United States. Keep in mind that these menu options change and that this list doesn't take into account cross contamination, shared oil, or well-trained employees.

Arby's: "Chopped side salad with potato cakes, please. Because there is almost nothing else I can eat here, and I'm dying for your curly fries."

Not surprisingly, Arby's isn't a vegan fast food mecca. In fact, like McDonald's (see below), this should probably be considered your last resort. However, if you don't mind a shared fryer, the actual ingredients in the curly fries are vegan. And they are very good.

Auntie Anne's Pretzels: Little-know vegan fast food fact: Auntie Anne's Original, Cinnamon Sugar, Sweet Almond, Garlic, Jalapeno, and Raisin pretzels can be veganized simply by ordering them specially made without the butter. Takes an extra five minutes, but it's worth it for a hot, soft pretzel on the go. Try dipping it into WayFare's new Dairy-Free Cheddar Dip. Thank me later.

Burger King: I hope you like fries, because that's one of the only things that's vegan at Burger King (their limited location veggie burger contains both eggs and dairy). Order up! "Large French fries, please, and hold everything else on your menu—except, double order, please, of the French toast sticks. I'll have it my way." There may be vegetables, toppings, and drinks you can also order, but otherwise, for now at least, Burger King isn't the greatest option for the traveling vegan (except those French toast sticks).

Carl's Jr. (and Hardee's): More brown food! "One order of the French fries, CrissCut fries, hash rounds, and hash-brown nuggets, please." All vegan. In the restaurant, there's an all-you-can-eat salad bar with a variety of vegetables and a three-bean salad. Surprisingly, you can also get the grits (which usually contains dairy). Kiss *those* grits, Flo.

Chick-fil-A: Unless you want one of their salads minus the chicken, the only cooked vegan options at Chick-fil-A are the Hash Browns (served only at breakfast) and the Waffle Potato Fries. You can also order a cool wrap and sub more veggies for the chicken. The BBQ sauce is vegan. They do serve a fresh Fruit Cup and Cinnamon Applesauce on the kid's menu, but you have to show ID proving you are ten.

Chipotle: The Burritos, Bowls, Tacos, and Salads at Chipotle Mexican Grill can be made vegan by ordering sofritas instead of meat. The tortillas, fajita vegetables, rice, beans, salsas, chips, and guacamole are all vegan, and they are also rolling out a braised tofu that's vegan. Note: their chipotle-honey vinaigrette is *not* vegan.

Denny's: You may not think of Denny's when you think of vegan food, but they serve Amy's brand burgers as the veggie patty for their vegetarian/ vegan Build Your Own Burger. The sesame seed and whole wheat buns are vegan, and you can even have fries on the side. This may be your best option if your local Denny's has the burger on their menu and you're craving retro diner food and a bottomless cup of joe.

Domino's: Domino's Pizza offers one vegan crust on their menu: the Thin Crust (the Gluten-Free crust contains honey). Top it with their Original Pizza Sauce and a bunch of veggies. Order a Garden Salad (hold the cheese) with balsamic or Italian dressing, and you've got a vegan meal your kids will love in under thirty minutes. Pro tip: Add shredded vegan mozzarella cheese and pop it back in the oven for ten minutes.

Dunkin' Donuts: Most of the bagels at DD are vegan. Order a toasted cinnamon raisin, cinnamon raisin bagel twist, everything, garlic, onion, plain, poppy seed, salt, or sesame, and top it with hash browns, an English muffin, a French roll, or a pretzel twist. Wash it all down with coffee cooled off with almond milk. Not much for nutritional variety, but there are plenty of vegan options to start your day off. If there were one food group I wish had more vegan options, it would be the donut food group.

Five Guys Burgers and Fries: Say, "Large fries, please." Five Guys hand-cut fries are served in an oil-soaked paper bag and will satisfy any salty craving. Keep in mind, however, that out of all the items on their menu (including their milkshakes), the large fries have more calories than anything else they serve. Get this: 1,200 whopping calories in a single order. They do offer a veggie sandwich (all their vegetables on a bun), but their bun contains dairy and eggs, so it's not vegan. Order your kids over 1,000 calories of French fries and a handful of sautéed onions like a good parent.

In-N-Out Burger: In-N-Out Burger may make the best fast food fries on the planet, and there is actually another vegan item that you're going to love. Just walk in and say, "One sandwich, no patty, no spread, and no cheese. Add the grilled onions, please." You'll get one of their secret menu items called "a veggie." The sandwich comes with lettuce, tomato, and onion on a fresh vegan bun and costs around $1.50. Trust me: order this with their amazing fries, and you're not going to miss the meat.

Jack in the Box: "One order of black beans, potato wedges, seasoned curly fries, and breakfast blueberry muffin oatmeal. And a drink cup big enough to bathe in." The list of vegan options at Jack in the Box is so limited, it's hard to imagine making a meal out of it, but they still get high marks for vegan curly fries (but I'll always love you most, Arby's curly fries).

Jimmy John's: Maybe, as a last resort, you can head to Jimmy John's for a "vegetarian unwich" without cheese or mayo. Basically, it's a veggie sub without the sub (their rolls aren't vegan). Add avocado spread for more flavor and top with oil and vinegar or Italian vinaigrette. All this and a bag of chips. Note: the owner of Jimmy John's is far from vegan, so maybe find another place.

KFC: Surprise! More fries! Order "One order of fries, side of green beans, corn on the cob without butter, and the KFC House Salad with the Golden Italian Light Dressing." It almost looks like a meal if you arrange everything in a strategic fashion before Instagramming it.

McDonald's: Lo and behold, the buns at McDonald's are actually vegan. Meanwhile, the fries aren't as the oil they're flavored with beef tallow. So, on the go, you can get a Big Mac bun loaded with lettuce, tomato, onion, and pickles, and just pretend that "after billions served," they finally ran out of beef patties. Not much else at McD's is vegan (unless your location still serves salads). Keep in mind, the bun contains enriched flour (which contains bleached wheat flour, malted barley flour, niacin, reduced iron, thiamin mononitrate, riboflavin, and folic acid), water, high fructose corn syrup and/or sugar, yeast, and soybean oil and/or canola oil. It contains 2 percent or less of salt, wheat gluten, calcium sulfate, calcium carbonate, ammonium sulfate, ammonium chloride, dough conditioners (may contain one or more of sodium stearoyl lactylate, datem, ascorbic acid, azodicarbonamide, mono and diglycerides, ethoxylated monoglycerides, monocalcium phosphate, enzymes, guar gum, and calcium peroxide), sorbic acid (preservative), calcium propionate and/or sodium propionate (preservatives), and soy lecithin. Some of these bun ingredients actually have side effects, so you may want to avoid McDonald's if at all possible.

Mid-2017, McDonald's announced they were going to release The McVegan, and everyone in Tampere, Finland (huh?), got excited for the monthlong trial. McDonald's claimed that if all went well, it could be rolled out around the world. We junk food and fast food vegans are understandably enthused.

Moe's Southwest Grill: Not unlike many Mexican fast food restaurants, Moe's offers a wide array of vegan options that include organic tofu, beans, tortillas, and rice. Order an Art Vandalay burrito without cheese, a Unanimous Decision taco without cheese, or the Instant Friend quesadilla or the nachos without cheese—and be sure to add the guacamole. Moe's also offers countless toppings and sides that are all vegan. Welcome to Moe's!

Panera: Panera Bread's Vegetarian Black Bean Soup is vegan. It has black beans cooked in a spicy vegetarian broth with onions, peppers, garlic, and cumin. Other vegetarian soups have dairy or honey, so be sure to check the ingredients. Have your soup with some ciabatta bread on the side. Obviously, Panera is a gamble, since most kids I know won't beg for black bean soup.

Papa John's Pizza: At this point on this list, you're getting very hungry. Pick up your phone and call Papa John's right now. I'll wait. Not so much for the thin crust pizza you're going to order with no cheese and tons of veggies, but rather for the garlic dipping sauce, which is vegan. Remember to ask for extra. Like, four extra.

Pizza Hut: I used to love going to Pizza Hut, so it's nice to know I can still order the Thin 'N Crispy or Hand-Tossed crust with the regular or sweet pizza sauce and "drag it through the garden." You'll be amazed at how satisfying a cheeseless pizza can be when it's loaded with vegetables. Turns out, the dessert crust at Pizza Hut is also vegan, so just navigate the vegan toppings to finish off your meal. Like Papa John's, have it to go and add your own vegan cheese at home.

Quiznos: Quiznos has a veggie sub you'll love. Order it "filled with guacamole, black olives, lettuce, tomatoes, red onions, and mushrooms, and no cheese." Ask for balsamic vinaigrette instead of red-wine vinaigrette. The vegan bread options include white or wheat, and there's also an herb wrap. Grab a side garden salad and some potato chips, and you'll forget you're vegan real fast.

Red Robin: Red Robin offers a Gourmet Vegan Burger that can be made vegan. It is topped tomato bruschetta salsa, avocado slices, and shredded romaine in a lettuce wrap. As if that's not enough to lure you in, they also offer vegan bottomless fries (to add to the size of our bottoms).

Ruby Tuesday's: Even back when I ate meat, I loved the salad bar at Ruby Tuesday's. I can still enjoy it now that I'm vegan. Their "Create Your Own Garden Bar" allows you to make a hefty vegan salad. There is spring mix, fresh greens, and lots of toppings like tomatoes, edamame, olives, green peas, and sunflower seeds. For dressings, choose from balsamic vinaigrette or olive oil and vinegar. You can also make a Veggie Trio Combo where you choose three side dishes. Fresh sides can include grilled asparagus, baked potato, grilled zucchini, steamed broccoli, fresh green beans, and roasted spaghetti squash. Just be sure to request that the veggies not be cooked in butter.

Sonic: "French fries, tots, sweet potato tots, and a side order of onion rings." Sonic. Home of the Vegan Brown Food. It's all these fried breaded potato dippables that remind me to always pack a to-go pack of Just Mayo. Just because.

Starbucks: The menu at Starbucks changes all the time. They've begun offering a variety of nondairy creamers for their coffee bar and specialty drinks. Keep in mind that many of the sugary flavors they use for their extra-fancy drinks aren't vegan. Your best bet at Starbucks is to ask someone what vegan options they have that day and to keep an eye on your barista to make sure she doesn't reach for the whole milk or whipped cream. As of October 2017, select South Florida locations will now stock vegan passionfruit cupcakes courtesy of local vegan bakery Bunnie Cakes.

Subway: Subway is always a savior when it comes to finding a vegan sandwich. The Veggie Delite has lots of veggies that you can choose, such as lettuce, tomatoes, green peppers, cucumbers, onions, and even guacamole (for that dreaded upcharge). Have it on their Italian, Hearty Italian, or Sourdough Bread. Top it with oil, vinegar, mustard, deli mustard, sweet onion sauce, or fat-free Italian dressing. If you're not up for a sandwich, order the Veggie Delite Salad and toss in a bag of chips or apple slices.

TCBY: Craving froyo? TCBY has you covered. They partnered with the soy milk brand Silk in 2013 to add dairy-free varieties to their menu, and many of their toppings are vegan. My personal weakness? Vanilla Silk frozen yogurt topped with peanuts and peanut butter sauce.

Taco Bell: Say, "Bean burrito and Chalupa fresco style, and sub the beans for meat!" Fresco means no dairy, and they'll put pico de gallo on it. By saying "fresco," you can pretty much eat the whole menu (except the

Doritos taco), though it might not hurt to also mention "no cheese or sour cream with vegan rice." Recommendations: bean burrito fresco, tostada fresco (already meatless), Mexican pizza. Add guacamole, since vegans add guacamole whenever it's available in spite of the dreaded upcharge.

Wendy's: If you go to Wendy's, you can order a Plain Baked Potato and a Garden Side Salad (the dinner salads have chicken and cheese). The salad has mixed greens, grape tomatoes, cucumbers, and bell peppers. Top it with Italian vinaigrette dressing but skip the croutons—they have dairy in them, of course, since what's a crouton without milk?

White Castle: Harold and Kumar approve of White Castle's vegan sliders (Dr. Praeger's brand). Order these bite-sized beauties plain or with a sweet Thai sauce. On January 14, 2014, *Time* magazine labeled the White Castle slider the most influential burger of all time. We can just pretend they meant the vegan burger.

It is essential to have patience and compassion when searching for vegan food options. After all, taking the extra time to save the life of a cow, pig, sheep, or fish is more important than eating one meal that you will forget about as soon as you swallow your last bite.
   Now . . . get traveling!

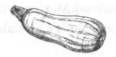

15

WHERE TO TURN: GETTING SUPPORT

"A good neighbor will babysit. A great neighbor will babysit twins."
—*Anonymous*

Where we live in Ithaca, New York, we've been very fortunate to be surrounded by many other vegans and countless other seasoned vegan parents. In fact, Ithaca has become somewhat of a hive of vegans. Vegans are everywhere. In fact, Ithaca has been ranked one of those most vegetarian-friendly cities in the country for a number of years, according to Priceonomics.com.

This small city, known for its universities and the home of Moosewood Restaurant, ranked third on a list of cities by Priceonomics.com for offering the most number of vegetarian restaurants per 100,000 people, with seventeen restaurants offering an ample selection of meat-free food. We never have issues eating out and finding vegan options. Amazingly, though, there are currently only two 100% vegan eateries.

This support network of vegans and veg-friendly folks has been there for us from day one, when we first went vegan, pre-kids, and today as we raise our own vegan kids. We host and attend regular potlucks, are invited to vegan drink events (which, of course, we cannot easily attend since we have two toddlers), and are fortunate enough to be able to reach out to an ever-expanding network of vegans whenever we have a question.

Most people aren't as lucky as we are and may feel alone in their journey. So, where do you turn for support when you feel like the only vegan in town?

Social media: Without a doubt, social media, and especially Facebook, offers countless opportunities to meet and engage with thousands of vegans. Just. Like. You. The level of support ranges from judgy and not-at-all-helpful to extremely supportive. Focus on the groups dedicated to raising vegan kids for now and post a "Hello, I'd love to connect," or "I am trying to raise my kids vegan but can't seem to find school lunch ideas that they like," and see how many other vegan parents out there extend a knowledgeable and compassionate hand. One group, Vegan Pregnancy and Parenting, has nearly 35,000 members who never hesitate to help.

Search for meetups in your region (as well as meetups for anywhere you plan to travel): Meetup.com lists many groups that have been formed around the country with all interests, and veganism (you may also search "animal rights") is usually quite active when it comes to hosting ongoing events. If you're lucky enough to live in New York City, there are over 13,000 members in that Meetup group (and the LA group has almost 6,000 members).

Join or form vegan clubs: Search your local area for any vegan clubs or the aforementioned more popular vegan drinks events. Meeting other vegans (even for adult events) will potentially help you connect with vegan parents while learning to navigate your own vegan journey. It's also an incredible feeling spending time with like-minded people.

Shop in the vegan sections of your local grocery store or food co-op: Stand in the vegan section of your local grocery store or co-op and wait, like a lion for a gazelle, to strike. Wait. Wait. And *BOOM*, she just grabbed the Beyond Burger! You found another vegan! Say "hi" without seeming like a stalker (which you are) and hope for the best (I'm sure it will work out . . . stalker).

Subscribe to email newsletters and mail lists: Many vegan and animal rights organizations offer vegan support guides and online vegan support courses and/or weekly emails. Download everything you can and sign up for anything that's free (these oftentimes contain manufacturer coupons for discounts on vegan food). These emails are rife with tips on going vegan and staying vegan, and it costs nothing to subscribe.

There are vegans everywhere; you just need to find them. Whether in real life or online. And once you do, you'll find support.

Of course, all of this leads back to why you bought this book in the first place. How do you raise vegan kids with, and without, outside support? Robyn Moore, who is raising her two kids vegan, has had her own set of challenges and obstacles, but for the most part she has found it to be easier than she thought it would be.

"I would first say that raising vegan kids is *much* easier than I thought it would be," Moore says. "Parenting in general is hard and full of many different challenges along the road, and being vegan is just one aspect. However, this lifestyle has the added benefit of allowing you to feel an inner peace and pride knowing you're raising kids according to deep values of compassion, responsibility, and integrity, with a heightened awareness for the animals we share our planet with. It's about accountability. It teaches kids to understand and recognize the effects that their choices have. Their choices are like a vote—either for something or against.

"There's not one formula for raising vegan kids or any kids; you just have to adapt and figure it out within your own family. That said, there is a huge and growing community of vegan families, and we should lean on each other and share advice, ideas, experiences, and inspiration. There are some really excellent, helpful websites and Facebook groups where people can share and ask questions about all things vegan kid–related, including nutrition, social events, activism, dealing with nonvegan friends and family, etc. I think those are really important, especially for parents living in isolated areas where they are the only vegan family in their town.

"Also, in my opinion, the best way to represent your vegan family is to let it play out naturally. By that, I mean when I meet new parents or attend school events, I don't immediately announce my veganism. I give people the chance to get to know me—and my kids—and by the time they find out we're vegan, they already know us and love our family. This means they're less likely to bring negative vegan stereotypes to the table and more likely to accommodate my kids' vegan lifestyle and be flexible and open. This is important (and often downplayed), especially if there's a chance these other parents/families will be in your life (and your kids'!) for many years. It sets the tone."

And, what about the skeptics? The ones who aren't necessarily supportive of your choice to raise your kids vegan?

"Very rarely do I have anyone question why I feed my kids a vegan diet," says Robin Fetter, mother of three. "What usually happens is the assumption that my kids eat healthier than theirs. Oftentimes, I have to remind them that there is a such thing as vegan junk food and that my kids like the vegan meats, cheeses, and treats as much as their kids would if they gave them a try! I have had my fair share of nonvegan families come to my home for a vegan meal, and I believe that alone answers all the myths they have about vegan nutrition—especially for kids. I like to think I gave them some solid ideas on what to serve their own kids the next time they want to provide them with a better option.

"I have a no-excuses, no-exceptions rule that no nonvegan food is allowed into my home, with the exception of infants who rely on formula. When people come over, I always make sure that there is more than enough food to go around, so there is never a question on what they are going to eat but rather what awesome vegan creation they are going to try next . . . and I swear I mean that in a *very* positive way! Most folks I know follow me on social media and already see the vegan food I eat. So coming over and not worrying about having to bring their own food is quite the treat for them."

Speaking of the influence of social media, I've personally posted hundreds of photos of vegan food porn featuring most of my recipes and culinary concoctions (mostly on Instagram: @anotherskepticalvegan). It has become the breakaway vegan acquisition platform for me as I promote the lifestyle. I get compliments, online and in person, about the food I post, which more and more people are willing to try.

So you've now committed to this lifestyle, you're working on your partner, and you've designed it to include your kids; but will it last?

"My confidence that my kids will stay vegan is pretty good," Robin continues. "My oldest is in first grade and has quite a bit of vegan knowledge under her belt. She isn't afraid to tell her friends at school why we shouldn't be eating animals. In fact, as we speak, I am waiting by my phone for an angry phone call from a teacher or parent about it! My two younger children know and understand the simpler message of veganism, which is 'we don't eat or use animals.' So when I tell them that a food contains a dead animal or that the elephant on TV doing tricks was stolen from his/her family, they want no part of it. I find that children 'get it' on a level that adults don't give them credit for.

"For example, I know several parents who have gone vegan but who kept their children on the same nonvegan path out of fear of social pressure or general resistance, but none of them ever sat down and had that conversation. They didn't even give the child a chance to process the information and understand veganism. Education is key. This doesn't mean finding the goriest animal cruelty video you can find, but you should break it down in a way your child will understand. You know your child better than anyone else, so choosing the context should be fairly easy. I like to think that this foundation of vegan values is something that will never leave my children, and hopefully it is something they can pass on to their own families."

The support is there if you seek it out. And the more support you get, the easier the transition will be. Hard things are put in our way not to stop us but to call out our courage and strength.

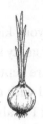

16

MY PARENTING MANTRA: SAFE, HAPPY, AND FED

"A father's goodness is higher than the mountain,
a mother's goodness deeper than the sea."
—*Japanese Proverb*

S ince the birth of my firstborn daughter, Gillian (from my first marriage), exactly twenty years ago, I've subscribed to one philosophy and one philosophy only when it comes to parenting. There are just three things you need to focus on when raising physically and mentally healthy kids. Provide a life for them where they know they will always be safe, happy, and fed.

Safe. Happy. Fed.

Just three words. Seems simple enough.

Safe. From the moment you first hold your newborn to the moment you accidentally drop them while unloading groceries; from the day you walk in on them making out in their bedroom when they're supposed to be at school to the tear-filled day you finally drop them off to college; and then from that tear-filled day (but for other reasons) they move *back* into your house for a year to every other cherished moment in the future, you're going to try to keep your kids safe. You're going to protect them from bad people and from falling off anything higher than a curb. You know that keeping your kids *safe* is the backbone to every other aspect of parenting. Their safety is priority, and, as a parent, you'll do anything to make sure they are kept out of harm's way.

Each night when I lie in bed with our two toddlers and they snuggle against me to hear the book I'm about to read, I can feel their own sense of security, knowing they are safe with their parents. This docile moment, of course, comes only after the two of them compete to see who can jump farthest across the room from the top of the bed.

Happy. Whatever your definition of happiness is, you're going to make sure your kids are happy. Smiling. Laughing. Every minute should be enjoyed and savored. Remember that happiness is a way of travel, not a destination. Give your happy kids choices that will in turn make them happy. Kids have very little control over their lives; they are constantly being told where to go, what to do, and what to eat. A little bit of control goes a long way toward feeling happy. You'll provide them with a life that allows them to find their own path and define their own happiness. And they will pursue happiness with tenacity. Safely.

In the long term, the basic elements that make children happy during their childhood seem to be the same ones that help them become happy adults: a secure relationship with their parents that provides the base to explore the world and develop self-confidence, all important factors in the recipe for happiness.

Fed. They need fuel to be safe and happy every day, and you're going to make sure you put the best, healthiest, and hopefully organic-iest possible foods into their growing bodies. You'll send them off to daycare, afterschool, elementary school, middle school, and high school with breakfast, even if it's something they have to finish on the school bus. You'll pack a healthy lunch for them or make sure that their school has healthy items on their menus. You'll take the time as often as your busy life will allow to make them a healthy, plant-based dinner.

Kids need real food to develop and thrive, and the more variety they are exposed to, the more foods they'll realize they enjoy and the better their eating habits will be.

If you focus on just these three words as you parent your littles every day, you'll have done everything in your own control to lay the groundwork for your healthy child's future. Over time, your kid will thank you for all of this (though it may take longer than you hope).

And, they'll especially thank you for choosing to raise them vegan. I'll never forget when our littlest one was born and I mentioned to a friend that we were planning on raising her vegan, like her older brother. The friend commented that they were impressed with our commitment. They knew how important it was to us and how much it would benefit our children.

They then went on to say that they wished they had done the same.

In our vegan (and also gluten-free) household, I do most of the cooking. What I cook is going to be vegan *and* nutritionally balanced, and both of our kids are getting everything they need from a plant-based diet. We're proud of what we've been able to accomplish in regard to their diets. Our kids are living their happy vegan lives and, ultimately, benefitting from our decision.

You might find yourself in a situation when well-meaning parents ask how can you raise, or "force," your kid to be vegan. Sherry Colb, whose two teen girls have been vegan for over a decade each, says, "In one form or another, this question arises with some frequency. The answer with respect to young children is that parents 'force' their children to do all sorts of things, both for their own good (e.g., brushing their teeth) and for the good of others (e.g., don't hit your friends). Because a vegan lifestyle is generally healthier than the standard American lifestyle, raising children as vegans is for their own good. Teaching children not to be speciesist is like teaching them not to be racist, sexist, or homophobic. If someone asked you 'how can you force your kids not to be white supremacists?' you would rightly think the questioner had a screw loose."

Asking that question about veganism is no different.

> "Let parents bequeath to their children not riches,
> but the spirit of reverence."
> —*Plato*

It's time to put to bed some assumptions about vegan parenting.

I may not be a professional parenting expert, but I'm not sure I even believe in the idea of "parenting experts." There are far too many variables. What I know is that I'm an engaged, imperfect parent and a passionate vegan. I'm also an experienced mapmaker, a cartoonist kids love, and a stumbling traveler. Like many of you, parenting is by far my boldest and most daring adventure.

Parenting vegan kids isn't extreme. The masses love to use the word *extreme* since it makes our "radical lifestyle" sound so much more exciting, as if we're a cult or a gang. A vegang. But is eating a variety of fresh vegetables, fruits, nuts, seeds, and grains really that radical? Is almond milk a sure sign of someone who has gone rogue?

Veganism is not about proselytizing or forcing our beliefs onto someone else. There wasn't a vegan meeting held to discuss how we are going to take over the world with the animals on our side. We didn't all decide to start reproducing so we could guarantee the survival of "the vegan." (Although this sounds like a great idea to me.)

Some of us just happen to have kids, that's all. And for those of us who do, why would we want to raise them any other way? An important part of parenting is passing down our own beliefs and values. Our kids just eat the same foods we eat; it's pretty simple.

It's precisely what omnivores are doing, but with animal welfare in mind. Raising vegan kids ensures they are healthy—in mind and in body.

"Aren't you worried that your kids might end up with a vitamin deficiency?" a friend, who suddenly becomes a nutritionist, will ask.

"They get everything they need from plants," I reply.

"Protein, though. You need to eat animals for protein," they will say.

"Really? Where do you think the animals you're eating get *their* protein?"

This usually calms them down.

"They're okay, I promise. We're looking after her, and I'm flattered you suddenly care so much about *our* kid's nutrition."

You must trust me: nothing is as important to us as our child's health and welfare. I wouldn't feed my children a diet that could put their health at risk. A vegan diet can provide all of the nutrients a growing child needs.

Plus, these are *our* lives. We're raising our two kids, and dog, vegan. Sometimes, we'll sit down with them and talk a little bit about why we eat the foods we do and why we don't always eat the same food as the other 94 percent of the population. And neither of these things are going to impact the lives outside of our family.

How popular is veganism becoming? Since my first book was released in 2017, the number of vegans worldwide grew from 2 to 6 percent. While this is still a very small segment of the population, at this rate, that 6 percent could become 18 percent in the next two years.

Omnivores can continue eating whatever they want; we're not criticizing their lifestyles simply by making different choices. We don't want them to feel upset, worried, or stressed about the fact that some of us choose to raise our kids vegan. Really, don't let it upset you; just think about something else.

One other thing: our kids aren't missing out, not even a little bit. Believe me when I say that our vegan kids don't cry each night into their bowls of sprouted mung beans. Our fridge and cupboards are filled with vegan cheeses, alt-milks, and enough vegan "junk food" to actually warrant *real* concern about their diets. Are they eating too much pizza, chocolate, crackers, and vegan sausages just like your kids? They're even eating bacon (made from plant-based ingredients, of course).

Our vegan lifestyle isn't that unusual. There are loads of us (and more are coming on board every day). Our friends are raising their kids vegans, and their friends are raising *their* kids vegan. And now, *you're* raising your kids vegan.

We're not doing this alone.

And, raising vegan kids isn't child abuse. This one will probably come as a shock to you, if you've been reading articles on Facebook about vegan babies dropping dead from malnutrition or parents who have been arrested for denying their kids the right foods.

In May 2017, a headline circulated in many vegan Facebook groups about a 2014 incident: "Malnourished baby dies after parents fed him insanely strict vegan diet." A seven-month-old baby in Belgium tragically died as a result of the strict diet his parents fed him, which exclusively consisted of gluten-free and lactose-free foods, as well as quinoa milk. According to the *New York Post*, the baby's parents self-diagnosed him with food allergies without ever consulting a doctor.

"The parents determined their own diagnosis that their child was gluten-intolerant and had a lactose allergy," public prosecutors said in court. "Not a single doctor had a dossier about Lucas and child protection services did not know about them."

Eventually, the pair did take the child to a homeopathic doctor, who insisted they take him to an actual hospital after observing the child's severe condition.

By the time they did, it was too late.

The seven-month-old weighed only nine and a half pounds when he died, half the size of the average baby his age.

This case had *nothing* to do with a vegan diet and everything to do with bad parenting. The headline was more than misleading, targeting vegans. Not only were these parents malnourishing their baby because of perceived allergies, they weren't making any effort to find alternative sources to keep him healthy, including, believe it or not, websites like OnlytheBreast.com that sells surplus human breast milk. Of course, going to the store and purchasing fortified gluten-free, vegan baby formula is a bit more convenient and also should have been considered.

Vegan kids *aren't*, the above incident aside, victims of child abuse. Child abuse is awful, and it's ridiculous to suggest that veganism, which represents the opposite of abuse, compares. Giving your kids dark chocolate instead of milk chocolate isn't *that* bad. They'll learn to live with it. I can't speak for every vegan child in the world, but the ones I personally know are safe, happy, and fed.

Parents raising their kids vegan is nothing new. It's tried and tested, and there are plenty of healthy lifelong vegans out there as living proof that a vegan upbringing is a pretty amazing thing.

Vegan parents are just like every other parent. We're parents who love our children—we just also happen to *really* love animals.

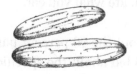

17

EATING ALL THE VEGGIES (AND MORE): RECIPES FOR THE LITTLE VEGANS

"Laughter is brightest in the place where the food is."
—*Irish Proverb*

It's incredible. You feed them and they poop; they poop more and then they grow. It's like magic. If the old saying "You are what you eat" ever had a place, it belongs in a vegan household with vegan kids. Nourish your little ones with bright, fun, colorful, and crunchy foods, and they will be bright, fun, colorful, and crunchy kids.

Crunchy Kids (band name).

History lesson: The actual phrase "You are what you eat" didn't emerge in English until sometime in the 1920s and '30s when nutritionist Victor Lindlahr, who was a strong believer in the idea that food controls health, developed the Catabolic Diet. That view gained some traction, and, ironically, considering the book you are holding, the earliest known printed example is from an advertisement for beef in a 1923 edition of the *Bridgeport Telegraph* for United Meat Markets:

Ninety per cent of the diseases known to man are caused by cheap foodstuffs. You are what you eat.

At least he was right about the 90 percent part of his marketing message; he was just misguided about the specific kinds of foods that are actually healthy.

As with any child, mealtime poses certain challenges for picky eaters. However, these proven, simple recipes are tasty and fun to make, and nine out of ten kids will love them. Make that tenth kid boxed vegan macaroni and cheese and store-bought vegan chicken nuggets dipped in vegan ranch dressing, and even *he* will be happy.

Eating vegan is a lot easier than you think. We've personally experimented with all the homemade and store-bought vegan foods you could imagine. To help with your own household, here are some of our easy tips for an instant vegan home:

Breakfast:
- Cereal. So many cereals are vegan, including Fruity Pebbles. We love Chex and Cheerios since they are also gluten-free.
- Plant-based milks. There are dozens to choose from; just find the one they love. They are delicious and nutritious, and the complete rundown is in chapter one.
- Vegan sausage and vegan bacon. These faux meats have come a long way, and our kids love them. Wrap the sausage up with vegan cheese in a tortilla, and heat and eat.
- Tofu scramble. As delicious as it is nutritious. Make your own homemade tofu scramble (be sure to always add a pinch of kala namak/black salt for a real egg taste) or try an easy store-bought brand like Amy's.
- Toast with peanut butter and jelly or vegan butter. Or, better yet, grill a PB&J *with* vegan butter for a hot take on the cold classic.
- Fruit. Cut it up into bite-sized pieces and serve with toothpicks for a fun morning treat. Pack the leftovers in their lunchboxes.

- Oatmeal sweetened with maple syrup. Our little girl devours this every time, usually asking for a second bowl.
- Pancakes and waffles with organic maple syrup. This is kind of a no-brainer.

Pro tip: Simply replace eggs with applesauce for all your sweet baked goods. Use plant-based milk and, voila—instant vegan pancakes, waffles, cupcakes, cakes, etc.

Lunch:
- Sandwiches and wraps. Filled with vegan cold cuts, meat, and vegan mayo, these are as good as their animal-based counterparts, and kids usually love them.
- Hummus wraps/hummus anything. Getting your kid to love hummus is the first rung in the vegan ladder. Next will be kale, followed by quinoa.
- Fruit. Cut it up into bite-sized pieces and serve with toothpicks as a fun lunchtime treat.
- Vegan yogurt. This has come a long way. Like the plant-based milks and ice creams (see below), there are too many to choose from, and you'll have to experiment with which ones your kids love best.

Pro tip: Buy a lidded bento box. Kids love eating with their hands, and the sectioned containers will allow you to give them a wide assortment of finger foods to enjoy. They're also very sturdy for the bus ride to and from school.

Dinner:
- Spaghetti or any pasta. Basil marinara, with or without vegan meatballs, is as easy as it gets.
- Garlic bread. Made with baguette, olive oil, and garlic, and toasted with vegan cheese.
- Tossed salad. Use a vegan ranch dressing or make your own, and top with shredded vegan parmesan cheese.

- Tacos. There is a sub-culture for vegan tacos that's about to explode. A favorite for almost everyone, they have become the cornerstone of vegan food.

Pro tip: Make a baked ziti, lasagna, or tofu bake casserole so you can divide your meals into portions that are the right size for each kid, as well as freeze portions for quick bites all week long.

Desserts:
- There are *so* many amazing vegan ice creams now that I don't dare to mention any here, for fear of inadvertently leaving one out or missing the dozen new ones that have been released since I wrote this paragraph. Many are from 100 percent vegan companies, but, noticing the popularity of veganism today, some ice cream companies you grew up on (Breyer's) are now also making vegan ice creams.
- Cake and cupcakes. Homemade or from a box, nothing beats a piece of cake. Except a donut. A vegan donut pretty much trumps every other vegan dessert.

Pro tip: Life's short; eat dessert first.

When I asked Physician's Committee for Responsible Medicine's (PCRM) Dr. Neal Barnard to contribute to this book, I was dancing around the subject of the difference between a *whole-foods, plant-based* diet and a *vegan* diet. I assured him that I knew the difference between the two, and that this book would try to balance the mindset that oil and salt and sugar are bad for you; that a vegan diet isn't always *that* healthy; and that the optimal diet for excellent health isn't vegan but rather plant-based.

Needless to say, I was more than delighted at his initial response to my concern.

"I would suggest not belaboring the idea that 'some vegan foods can be unhealthy.' True, there are sugary vegan foods nowadays, but we don't want to suggest that vegans eat worse than people who include meat, dairy, etc., in their diets." Dr. Barnard was finally saying what I've always wanted someone to say to me since I went vegan. "Going to a vegan diet is a good move, and once one has done that, one can make further improvements."

So much of what you already eat and what you already feed your family is vegan. Start there. Feed them all the vegan foods, and, as the good doctor says, you'll soon find yourself eating healthier as part of the process.

Vegan kitchen basics to keep your kids fueled:
In addition to popular and easy-to-find staples that have been vegan all along (rice, pasta, spices, most bread, etc.), there are a few ingredients you'll always want on hand before you've truly become your kid's vegan short-order cook. Of course, buy organic when you can (avoid GMOs if you want), and if possible join your local CSA to get the freshest fruits and vegetables possible. In my opinion, the ingredients listed here are a requirement—a rite of passage—for vegan cooking. Many of these will help your kid forget they were ever meat eaters.

Potatoes: You might have guessed that these would be at the top of this list. Any kind, any size. Always have them on hand to create a tasty side dish or potato salad, whether baked, mashed, or fried. Potatoes are inexpensive and easy to prepare. There are so many variations of preparing potatoes that there are entire cookbooks dedicated to this versatile root vegetable.

Nutritional yeast (nooch): This magical golden dust adds a nutty, almost cheesy, flavor to many recipes and is used in everything from tofu scramble to macaroni and cheese. It can be purchased online or at nearly every well-stocked grocery. It's also an excellent source of that elusive B12 you've been hearing all about. (Warning: while most popular brands of nooch are fortified with B12, sometimes the nooch you buy in bulk is not. Read the label.) We try to add a dash of nooch to everything we make.

Better than Bouillon (vegan version): Or any other organic vegetable-based bouillon. This is great for sautéing vegetables without oil, rehydrating textured vegetable protein (TVP), or making a super simple risotto that kids *actually* love.

Himalayan sea salt: Or any sea salt you can find. While most advocates for a whole-food, plant-based diet usually avoid added salt and oil, it's nice to have this and a good pepper mill on hand to bring out the flavors in your cooking. Salt is a flavor enhancer and should always be used sparingly. Unless on French fries.

Smoked paprika: I love this simple spice that I add to almost all of my meaty dishes. Add a dash to any recipe to give it that lumberjack flavor without having to swing an ax. It also adds a red color to some of the faux meat recipes you're about to take on. There are many variations on smoked spices you can try, and I recommend any of these over liquid smoke.

Rice: White, brown, long grain, short grain, risotto (Arborio). Rice serves as an excellent foundation, or side, for many vegan meals. The Korean dish bibimbap is a rice bowl covered in chopped up veggies that kids will love. Add wheat-free tamari (soy sauce) or spicy gochujang (available vegan), and get creative with this simple one-bowl meal.

Wheat-free tamari: This is the gluten-free version of soy sauce, and I always recommend that people become accustomed to buying this instead of regular soy sauce. It tastes the same, and if you find out your partner is gluten-intolerant (like I did), you'll score extra points when you pull this out. You can also use Bragg's Liquid Aminos, a similar product in desperate need of a new name. "Hey, kids! You want some liquid aminos for your vegan sushi?" See what I mean?

Beans: Where do I begin with beans? They are so important and versatile that all I can say is 1) dried beans take longer to make and may not be worth the extra effort; 2) canned beans should be organic and in a

PBA-free lined can. Adzuki, black, chickpea, fava, kidney, lentil, navy, pinto, or white. Buy all the beans; they are the musical fruit, after all.

Pasta (preferably gluten-free, for the same reasons mentioned): As a side or main dish, you could literally survive off a nice brown rice pasta and a million different sauces (with vegetable toppings). A simple Alfredo sauce will make you feel guilty about eating all the pasta, as well as a meat-free bolognese that uses beans. Buy all the beans.

Nuts: Raw cashews and almonds are great for making creams and dairy-free milks. Peanuts are great (I especially love Linus), and a lot of people add walnuts to bean burgers to make them meatier. Keep in mind that many kids (and adults) have specific nut allergies, especially when you're preparing meals for potlucks or other occasions, so it's good to ask first if you're making something for someone else.

Texturized vegetable protein (TVP): Texturized vegetable protein, also known as textured soy protein, soy meat, or soy chunks, is a defatted soy flour product, a by-product of extracting soybean oil. It is often used as a meat replacement or meat extender. It is quick to cook, with a protein content far greater than that which comes from animal meat. There are also variations such as Butler Soy Curls that add incredible taste, texture, and protein to any meal (think tacos).

Oil and vinegar: Again, avoid oil as much as you can, but if you're going to use it (I do), use extra virgin olive oil, high-heat sesame oil, or coconut oil. Vinegars come in an amazingly delicious array of flavors, and a simple splash added to any salad does wonders. Your kids are sure to love the vinegars that are infused with fruit flavors.

Maple syrup or brown rice syrup: Excellent sweeteners that aren't pure sugar. For a sugar substitute, try evaporated cane juice, which is a fancy name for "more natural" sugar. Agave nectar is another sweetener we use, especially in lemonade.

Lemons and limes: While I don't mention these in most of the recipes in this book, squeezing a fresh lemon or lime onto pretty much anything adds a burst of freshness that tastes fantastic (the same can be said for many fresh herbs like basil, parsley, or mint). Plus, it's a laugh riot giving a baby a slice of lemon to chew on.

Sauces: Always have the pantry or fridge filled with your favorite barbecue sauces, marinades, tomato sauces, and marinaras, plus that important full bottle of Sriracha for the more adventuresome kids.

Spices: Have as many or as few spices on hand as you like, but it's always best to have the basics around. Most of the minimally required spices are covered in the recipes here. By all means, load up your spice rack with classics like Simon and Garfunkel's "Parsley, Sage, Rosemary, and Thyme."

Recipes:
Finally! Here is the list of vegan recipes, and they're in alphabetical order! I've included one recipe for each letter of the alphabet, so you can try a new snack every day for twenty-six days, and then start over. You can also use this list as a song, sung to the tune of "You Are My Sunshine," to remind your little vegans that there is plenty to eat. You're welcome.

ANTS ON A LOG

Ingredients:
1 stalk of celery
½ cup organic peanut butter
Few dozen raisins
½ cup vegan dark chocolate chips

A classic and simple recipe. Wash celery stalk and cut into 6-inch lengths. Fill the gutter with peanut butter and adorn the top with a row of raisins. So simple and fun to make. And if you want to add a bonus for your kids, you'll use dark chocolate chips.

BANANA SUSHI

Ingredients:
1 banana
1 Tbsp favorite nut butter (peanut or almond)
¼ cup crushed peanuts
1 Tbsp sesame seeds
¼ cup vegan rainbow sprinkles
1 Tbsp Hershey's chocolate syrup

Peel the banana and cut lengthwise. Flat side up, spread on nut butter. Sprinkle on optional toppings (nuts, seeds, rainbow sprinkles) and press them lightly into the nut butter to ensure that they will stick. Using a sharp knife, evenly slice the banana into "sushi" pieces. Enjoy right away by dipping into Hershey's chocolate syrup, or transfer onto a baking sheet and freeze for later.

CHEESY MACARONI

Ingredients:

1 12 oz. bag elbow macaroni

2 cups unsweetened non-dairy milk

1 12 oz. bag shredded vegan cheddar cheese

¼ cup nutritional yeast

¼ cup bread crumbs or potato chips (optional)

When people ask how we make such amazing vegan macaroni and cheese, I always tell them we make it the exact same way you make the dairy version; we just use vegan ingredients. Cook your elbow pasta according to the directions, drain, and set aside. In large, deep pan, slowly heat up 2 cups unsweetened plant-based milk until just bubbly. Slowly add one full bag of shredded vegan cheese and ¼ cup nutritional yeast until a creamy sauce is formed. Stir in your cooked pasta and enjoy. Or, you can transfer to a baking dish and top with breadcrumbs or crumbled up potato chips and bake for twenty minutes at 400 degrees.

DONUT APPLES

Ingredients:

6 large apples

½ cup Enjoy Life dark chocolate chips

¼ cup vegan rainbow sprinkles

Cut apples into the shape of donuts (slice sideways and then core with a shotglass). Melt chocolate chips in double boiler or simply microwave in a bowl for 3–5 minutes, stirring halfway through. Dunk half of the apples into the melted chocolate and sprinkles, and refrigerate for a few hours. They're at least half healthy.

EDAMAME

Ingredients:
Bag of frozen or fresh edamame
Sprinkle of sea salt

These are actually soybeans. They are a delicious and nutritious snack and, surprisingly, most kids love them. Add a little sea salt or just pop in your little kids' mouths from across the room. Score extra points for each bean that actually makes it into their mouths.

FRUIT KEBABS

Ingredients:
Large bunch red or green grapes
1 cup fresh blueberries
1 cup sliced strawberries
2 sliced bananas
Wooden skewers

Everything's more fun when it's eaten off a skewer! Slide grapes, blueberries, sliced strawberries, sliced bananas, etc., onto a wooden skewer. Quarter the larger pieces of fruit for younger children. For older children, ask them to construct the kebabs in the order of the colors of the rainbow.

GARBANZO BEANS

Ingredients:

One 15 oz. can organic
    garbanzo beans (chickpeas)*
1 Tbsp olive oil

Pinch of sea salt
½ tsp garlic powder

Garbanzo beans are packed with protein. They are delicious when baked or air-fried. Drain and rinse one can of garbanzos and dry between two paper towels. Toss in a bowl with a small amount of olive oil, salt, and garlic powder. Bake at 450 degrees for 30–40 minutes until crispy.

*Pro tip: Save the liquid! The world of garbanzo beans changed forever when some genius decided to save the liquid from the can and whip it up with a high-speed mixer to reveal its frothy, whipped creaminess! Add some sugar and a little vanilla, and refrigerate for a pie topping. Google "aquafaba recipes" for even more exciting garbanzo bean recipes.

HUMMUS AND CRACKERS (OR CUKES)

Ingredients:

One 15 oz. can organic garbanzo
    beans
3 Tbsp olive oil
3 Tbsp tahini
½ lemon

One clove garlic
Salt
Pepper
Crackers or cucumbers, to serve

Making homemade hummus is so simple with your high-speed blender or food processor. Combine in your blender the garbanzo beans (roughly 2 cups drained) with the olive oil and tahini. Squeeze in lemon juice and add a small clove of garlic. Blend until smooth. Add salt and pepper to taste. Serve with crackers or sliced cucumbers.

ICE POPS

Ingredients:
Organic fruit juice of your choice
Variety of fresh cut fruits (pineapple, strawberries, etc.)

At most home stores, you can purchase an ice pop kit—plastic containers with snap-on lids that have a stick and a handle for making popsicles. Fill each with some fruit juice and sliced fruit (we like strawberries), making sure you leave a little room at the top for when it freezes. Freeze overnight and enjoy the next day! Experiment with different juices and other fruit pieces.

JELL-O (VEGANIZED)

Ingredients:
Store-bought vegan Jell-O
Sliced fresh fruit pieces (optional)

There is a vegan Jell-O out there! It's prepared exactly like the original version (which, by the way, contains horse hooves because of the gelatin). Make this with the added fruit slices you loved as a kid.

KALE CHIPS

Ingredients:
One bunch of kale
½ tsp olive oil
Pinch of sea salt
¼ cup nutritional yeast (optional)
Spices (optional)

You will be very surprised at how quickly your kids will devour these kale chips. Thoroughly wash a bunch of kale. De-stem and dry on a clean dishtowel before tearing into bite-size pieces. Toss with olive oil, a little salt, and some nutritional yeast or spices (optional). Place on cookie sheet covered with parchment paper, and bake at 300 degrees for about 10 minutes. Enjoy!

LEMONADE

Ingredients:
12 lemons
8 cups water
¼ cup agave nectar (or other sweetener)

Ideally, you'll already have some sort of lemon juicer on hand; if not, you're going to get very tired squeezing out the juice of twelve lemons into a large pitcher (try catching all the seeds). Add 8 cups of water and ¼ cup of agave nectar, and stir. Last time I made this, Cooper thought he was being funny by drinking straight-up the lemon juice we had just squeezed. Of course, he took one sip and spit it all back into the juice we were hoping to drink.

LIQUID GOLD

I just had to add another "L" to make sure this super simple and tasty recipe made it into this book. This is a variation on the original recipe by our friends Lewis and Priscilla, which appears in their *Great Life Cookbook* (an excellent source for whole-foods, plant-based recipes for larger families).

Ingredients:
1 large butternut squash
Three medium white onions
Salted water
¼ cup agave nectar (or maple syrup)
Pinch of salt

Peel and dice the butternut squash into 2-inch cubes. Peel and rough cut the onions. Bring to boil 3 quarts of salted water and add the onions. Let boil for five minutes, and then add the cubed squash. Boil until squash is fork-tender (falls apart). Carefully strain and place into a high-speed blender. Blend on high until a thick soup is formed. Add the agave nectar and blend for another minute. Salt to taste. Perfect as soup, baby food, or sauce on top of rice.

MANGO DICES

Ingredients:
A couple ripe mangoes

Stand the mango on your cutting board, stem end down, and hold. Place your knife about ¼ inch from the widest center line and cut down through the mango. Flip the mango around and repeat this cut on the other side. The resulting ovals of mango flesh are known as the "cheeks." What's left in the middle is mostly the mango seed.

Cut parallel slices into the flesh of the mango cheeks, being careful not to cut through the skin. Turn the mango cheek around and cut another set of parallel slices to make a checkerboard pattern.

Here's where you can choose your favorite method. Either "Slice and Scoop"—scoop the mango slices out of the mango skin using a large spoon—or "Inside Out"—turn the scored mango cheek inside out by pushing the skin up from underneath and scrape the mango chunks off of the skin with a knife or spoon. Or, eat with a toothpick right off the mango!

MINI PIZZAS

Ingredients:
6 vegan English muffins
½ cup favorite vegan tomato sauce
12 oz. bag shredded vegan
   mozzarella

Favorite vegan pizza toppings or
   cut vegetables

We all remember these from our childhood. Kids love making their own pizzas. Toast vegan English Muffins (Thomas' are not vegan, but Trader Joe's, Aldi, and many store brands are) and spread jarred pizza sauce on top. Add vegan mozzarella and any other toppings you like. Broil until the cheese melts.

NUTTY NOODLES

Ingredients:

5 Tbsp hot water	2 tsp lemon juice
3 Tbsp peanut butter	3 quarts water
2 Tbsp soy sauce or tamari	Rice noodles

Peanut sauce is so simple to make, and it tastes delicious over quick-cooking rice noodles. Mix 5 Tbsp hot water with peanut butter, soy sauce or tamari, and lemon juice. Microwave for 30 seconds. Bring 3 more quarts of water to a boil and add rice noodles. Cook for 3–4 minutes and drain. Top with sauce.

OLIVE YOU

Ingredients:
Olives!

Olives are such a great snack. Children love putting them on the ends of their fingers. There's no real recipe here. Just look for a Mediterranean bar the next time you're shopping and load up a container with a variety of olives of different sizes and colors, and let your kids keep track of which ones they love the best (then, buy those next time).

POPCORN

Ingredients:
Popcorn
Coconut oil
¼ cup nutritional yeast
Pinch of sea salt

Popcorn can be popped ahead of time and sealed into Ziploc baggies. Try popping it with coconut oil (according to the package instructions) and sprinkle with nutritional yeast and sea salt for added nutrition and flavor.

QUINOA PUDDING

Ingredients:
1 cup cooked organic quinoa
Dash of cinnamon
¼ cup almond milk
Chopped up apple (optional)

Quinoa with cinnamon and almond milk is delicious served as a hot breakfast cereal. Prepare cup of quinoa according to the package directions. Make it ahead of time, and serve it in the morning.

ROASTED SWEET CHICKPEAS

Ingredients:

1 can of chickpeas	½ tsp cinnamon
½ Tbsp olive oil	⅛ tsp nutmeg
1 Tbsp maple syrup	⅛ tsp fine sea salt

A variation on the savory baked garbanzo beans (page 172), these sweet treats pack a protein-filled punch. Drain and rinse chickpeas and pour into a lightly greased nonstick pan set over low heat. Cook for a good 20 minutes, constantly stirring. Once the chickpeas begin to brown, add olive oil, maple syrup, cinnamon, nutmeg, and fine sea salt, and cook for an additional 10 minutes. Allow to cool before snacking.

SEAWEED SNACKS ROLLED AROUND RICE

Ingredients:
1 cup prepared white rice
1 6 oz. package of seaweed snacks (nori)

Prepare the white rice according to the package instructions. Let cool for 20–30 minutes. Take one sheet each of the seaweed snack and cover with a thin layer of rice. Roll seaweed over the rice and feed to your kids!

TRAIL MIX

Ingredients:

½ cup mini pretzels

¼ cup dark chocolate chips

¼ cup almonds or cashews

¼ cup raisins or craisins

1/8 cup sunflower seeds

1/8 cup favorite dried fruit (I love pineapple)

This is a great to-go snack, and the varieties are endless. Mix pretzels, dark chocolate chips, nuts, raisins, sunflower seeds, and dried fruit in large bowl and portion out into snack bags for a simple school or travel snack. The mix can be made to accommodate many dietary preferences.

UMAMI ALMONDS

Ingredients:

16 oz. raw almonds

¼ cup tamari or soy sauce

Umami is the fifth taste in the sweet, salty, bitter, and sour taste categories. It is often described as rich and savory. Soy sauce or its gluten-free equivalent, tamari, adds an umami flavor to this simple nut recipe. Bake raw almonds on a parchment-lined baking sheet for 10 minutes at 300 degrees. Remove from the oven and mix with tamari or soy sauce. Let soak for 20 minutes before putting back into the oven for 20 minutes. Let the almonds cool completely; they will become firmer as they cool.

VANILLA SMOOTHIE

Ingredients:
1 banana, frozen
2 cups sweetened plant-based milk
1 Tbsp vanilla

Place one frozen banana in a blender with plant-based milk. Add vanilla extract and blend until very smooth (1 minute on high).

WATERMELON BURGERS

Ingredients:
Marinade:
¼ cup wheat-free tamari (soy sauce)
2 Tbsp vegan BBQ sauce (most are already vegan)
1 Tbsp smoked paprika
Pinch of sea salt
2 Tbsp nutritional yeast
2 Tbsp olive oil

Burger:
1 large watermelon

Toppings:
Favorite vegan cheese
Lettuce, tomato, onion (optional)

Whisk all ingredients for the marinade in flat-bottom bowl or 8-inch casserole dish, and set aside. Slice your watermelon into 1-inch slices and then punch them out with a glass (so they are round). Marinate overnight in a casserole dish in the sauce, turning once after a few hours. Pan fry or grill the watermelon patties the next day, and serve topped with melted vegan cheese, lettuce, tomato, and ketchup. Like carrot dogs, your kids could eat these endlessly since they are made out of fruit.

XTRA ENERGY COOKIES

Ingredients:
2 bananas, the riper the better
1 cup oatmeal
Mini dark chocolate chips (optional)

Okay, that's pushing it for the letter X, but trust me, this recipe is worth it since you know your kids *need* more energy. Mash the bananas and mix with oatmeal. Add dark chocolate chips, if you like. Drop 2 Tbsp of the mixture onto a cookie sheet lined with parchment paper and bake at 350 degrees for 30 minutes.

YAM FRIES

Ingredients:
2 large/long yams
1 Tbsp olive oil
Pinch of sea salt
Ketchup or vegan ranch dressing, to serve

Are sweet potatoes the same as yams? They are, for this recipe. Peel your yams and carefully cut them into the shape of fries (roughly ½-inch thick and 5–6 inches long). In a large bowl, toss with a little olive oil and sea salt. Spread in one layer on a cookie sheet and bake at 375 degrees for 30 minutes, turning them over after 15 minutes. Serve with ketchup or vegan ranch dressing.

ZUCCHINI CHIPS

Ingredients:
1 zucchini
1 cup plant-based milk
2 cups flour
¼ cup nutritional yeast
1 cup bread crumbs

Chips are popular with kids no matter what they're made from! Slice a zucchini into thin slices and dip in plant-based milk. Mix flour with nutritional yeast in a bowl and coat zucchini chips. Dip again in the milk and then coat with bread crumbs. Place on a baking sheet covered with parchment paper and bake at 350 degrees for 15 minutes or until browned.

Vegan alternatives:
Today, there is a delicious vegan version of everything you could ever want to feed your kids. Some are more successful than others in mimicking the original, and we've pretty much tried every one at some point along the way. While this list is a great starting point and many are excellent transitional foods, by the time you've finished reading this book (and you're almost there now), you'll find more.

The latest and most innovative new products are launched every year at the weekend-long Natural Products Expo (ExpoWest and ExpoEast) in Anaheim, California, and Baltimore, Maryland, respectively. These are the world's largest shows of their kind, so if you ever have reason or ability to attend, it's worth it. All the major vegan and plant-based food companies are in attendance, and each attempts to one-up the other for innovative new vegan foods. And, if you can get press or blogger credentials, you get to sample them all. It's not an event for the kids, though.

Please note: Not all of the foods listed here are available nationwide or in certain retail outlets. However, availability in the past few years has expanded into some very unexpected places. Walmart, Target, Aldi, and even some dollar stores across the country are stocking their shelves with vegan goodies. Also, if you have a food co-op near you, they will often special-order items (like the time we had them order us a case of Sol Cuisine breakfast patties even though they stopped carrying them).

All of these foods are certified vegan and get the Lindstrom family stamp of approval:

Meat: Beyond Meat, Gardein, Sol Cuisine, Trader Joe's Soy Chorizo, Boca, Field Roast, and Tofurky are the most popular and readily-available brands.

Milk: Silk (makes soy, almond, and cashew), Pacific Foods, So Delicious, Ripple, and WestSoy are the ones we have on hand at all times. Our kids love the sweetened vanilla varieties the best (see chapter one).

Cheese: Chao, Follow Your Heart, Violife, Miyoko's Kitchen, Daiya, and Kite Hill have all been kid-approved for meltability and yumminess.

Eggs: Follow Your Heart's VeganEgg, The Vegg, and Ener-G brands are the three we have in our house, but we also use applesauce in place of eggs when baking.*

Honey (sweeteners): Bee Free Honee, maple syrup, brown rice syrup, and agave nectar all do the trick and leave the bees alone.

Condiments: Just Mayo, Just Ranch, Just Caesar, Just Thousand Islands, Follow Your Heart Vegenaise, Chipotle Vegenaise, and Tofutti sour cream and cream cheese are all amazing. And, of course, ketchup and mustard are already vegan.

*Pro tip: Did you know you can buy almost any cake mix on the market and use applesauce for eggs, alt-milk for milk, and vegan butter for butter? They'll turn out just as delicious. Combine that with frosting whipped up with powdered sugar, alt-milk, and vegan butter (colored with beet juice or turmeric), and you can start making muffins, cupcakes, and cakes like a pro.

Appliances and gadgets:
There are certain gadgets, tools, and appliances you should have in your kitchen to help you keep your vegan kids fed. Some are required and others are recommended, and we use all in our home.

- Vitamix (or any other high-speed blender)
- Immersion blender
- Rice cooker/vegetable steamer
- Slow cooker/Crock-Pot
- Mixer (hand or stand)
- Food processor or mini food chopper
- Teppanyaki grill (optional, but we love ours)
- Air fryer (optional, but oh-so-good; see below)

JL Fields is a culinary instructor, author of *The Vegan Air Fryer* and *Vegan Pressure Cooking,* and co-author of *The Main Street Vegan Cooking Academy Cookbook* and *Vegan for Her.* When I told JL I was looking for the best all-around appliance for the kitchen when cooking for vegan kids, she immediately recommended the Air Fryer. And she knows what she's talking about; she literally wrote the book.

"I'm known for keeping the making and eating of vegan food 'real,'" JL says. "No need to complicate the uncomplicated, am I right? One of the ways I keep cooking easy is to use gadgets to speed things along. My two favorites are a pressure cooker (you might know it as an Instant Pot) and an air fryer.

"Air frying is *magical.* Essentially, you're using a small countertop device to push hot air rapidly around food to make it crispy, using little to no oil. The lower oil aspect is nice because it means you can enjoy familiar fried foods without all the mess and, bonus, a little less fat. But what I really love about these devices is that you can cook food super fast. And your kids can get involved, too. Frozen vegan food can cook up in about eight minutes: French fries, tater tots, frozen burritos, gardein tenders, Tofurky pockets, mini pizzas, you name it."

Just search "vegan air fryer" on Google or Pinterest and you'll see all the amazing things parents are doing in this countertop appliance.

"In addition to quickly heating frozen foods, you can make easy homemade treats and meals, too," JL continues. "Slice up some potatoes and have them ready to roll for quick home-cooked fries or potato chips. Make or purchase pizza dough and get into the kitchen with your kids to dress up that pizza with tomato sauce, their favorite vegan meat and veggies, and maybe even a little vegan cheese. Those mini pizzas cook up in the air fryer in ten minutes."

Homemade food that is fun and quick to air fry:
- Doughnut holes: 8 minutes
- Grilled cheese sandwiches: 5 minutes
- Fried tofu nuggets: 10–15 minutes
- Chimichangas (air-fried burritos): 10–12 minutes
- Fried mushrooms: 7 minutes
- Roasted vegetables: 10–12 minutes
- Vegan corndogs: 12 minutes
- Single serving cookie: 8 minutes

"While air fryers can get hot, the parents I work with say that with proper education and supervision, their children are self-sufficient with the air fryer," JL adds. "They use wood spoons or silicone tongs to remove food, or they know to simply remove the air fryer basket by the handle and dump food directly on a plate.

"So, if you're looking for a cooking shortcut to create vegan food that your kids will love—and can even prepare on their own—the air fryer will come to the rescue!"

Other gadgets and tools for your vegan kitchen:
- Nonstick frying pan
- Heat-rated silicone spatulas (small and large)
- Measuring spoons and cups
- Sharp knife set
- Whisks
- Locking tongs
- Strainer/colander
- Microplane grater
- Potato/vegetable peeler
- Mandoline slicer
- Wooden spoons
- Citrus juicer (manual or electric)
- Tofu press

18

RESOURCES: MOVIES, BOOKS, WEBSITES, ROAD TRIPPING, AND MORE

"Don't ever stumble over what's behind you.
Neither trip over tomorrow. Just focus on today."
—*Anonymous*

Reading to your kids is one of life's greatest pleasures. I should know, since I do it upwards of ten times each night as we put down our two little (jumpy-jumpy) angels. Just when you think they're down . . . jump!

Reading children's stories as a vegan, however, poses more of a creative challenge than you might expect. Films and TV are just as difficult to manage. Many of the classics are steeped in so much cultural history and tradition about meat, milk, and eggs, and most authors naturally carry these unvegan messages into their own recent works. Which is why we often work on rewrites of the classics.

Little Miss Muffet

Little Miss Muffet sat on her tuffet
Eating her curds and whey

When along came a spider
And sat down beside her
And frightened Miss Muffet away. Reminding her that a dairy-based diet increases her risk of breast, lymphoid, and, remarkably, lung cancers. And contributes to the development of colic, allergies and digestive problems, and heart disease.

And, by supporting the dairy industry, she is contributing to the rape and mistreatment of dairy cows and the slaughtering of male calves for veal.

That afternoon, Little Miss Muffet went vegan.

Maybe not *this* rewrite, but you get the picture.

While you can certainly edit fairy tales and books with as much detail as you like as you go along (this is what we do since our kids can't read and we can pretty much make up everything), there are many amazing vegan books and films available for kids, created by many amazingly talented vegans.

"There are now a number of kids' books about veganism, including my favorite—Ruby Roth books. *Vegan Is Love* is a wonderful book." Sherry Colb says. (Sherry has been kind enough to give our family hand-me-down vegan books from her own children.) "There are also films that capture this message to a greater or lesser extent. I remember once reading the first few lines of *Charlotte's Web* to one of my girls and getting the delighted reaction, 'Hey! That's a vegan book.' Even though it is not, there are themes that can be understood within a vegan framework (for example, Fern's desire—and then Charlotte's plan—to save Wilbur's life from slaughter). A lot of what veganism education involves is generalizing from stories of individual animals (like Wilbur) and the value that we place on their lives to the lives of other animals just like them who also deserve to live."

Robin Fetter has her own perspective on reading books to her young vegans.

"I have children who are learning to read, so oftentimes changing a word as I read can be a disservice. I usually avoid books that have nonvegan items for that very reason. Maybe later on when they have a better grasp of literacy and can connect that nonvegan word with animal cruelty, I might be able to reintroduce those books. But for now, I tend to read the books to myself first before reading them to my kids or having my kids read the books to me. Luckily, there are quite a few vegan children's authors, and that number seems to be growing by the day. My kids prefer those books above anything else because it's usually about things they are familiar with."

Favorite books with a vegan message from our own vegan home library:
And Here's to You by David Elliott (Candlewick Press)

From the book that states, "Here's to the birds and the bears and the bugs and all the other critters we share the air with," David Elliott's infectiously joyful poem and Randy Cecil's colorful, brilliant, amusing artwork invite us to celebrate the world's vast diversity—and feel pretty happy with our place in it, too.

Benny Brontosaurus Goes to a Party by L. Farnsworth (SK Publishing)

I read this book often to our son. He was intensely interested in finding out how this fearful dinosaur would do with his meat-eating friends. I think it helps him to feel proud of his vegan diet. Did you know that in real life, the brontosaurus (and many other massive dinosaurs) was vegan? Yep. Highly recommended.

Caterpillar Dreams by Clive McFarland (HarperCollins)

The protagonist of this book—written and illustrated by Clive McFarland—is a teeny caterpillar who dreams of flying and exploring the world outside of the garden where he lives. He works hard to achieve his dream. Then, something miraculous happens, and everything for which he had hoped comes true. This sweet book offers subtle lessons on the importance of dreams, the value of friends, and the amazing things that life can bring.

Charlotte's Web by E. B. White (Harper and Brothers)

This timeless novel tells the story of a pig named Wilbur and his friendship with a barn spider named Charlotte. When Wilbur is in danger of being slaughtered by the farmer, Charlotte writes messages praising Wilbur (such as "Some Pig" and "Terrific") in her web in order to persuade the farmer to let him live. The films are just as fun to watch with the kids.

Dave Loves Chickens by Carlos Patiño (Vegan Publishers LLC)

You can tell this will be a fun book by the brightly colored illustration on the cover, featuring Dave, an alien embracing two chickens. Colorful and upbeat, *Dave Loves Chickens* still comes with a serious message and valuable information for children about our friends, a.k.a. the chickens. "As you and I and Dave will agree," writes author and illustrator Carlos Patiño, "chickens are great, and they don't belong on your plate."

Does a Kangaroo Have a Mother, Too? by Eric Carle (HarperCollins)

This was a favorite of mine when the kids were very little. It's a board book that helps kids see similarities between themselves and other animals by pointing out that every animal has a mother, and every mother loves her babies. Each page features a different animal with passages like, "Does a kangaroo have a mother, too? Yes, a kangaroo has a mother, just like me and you."

Eating the Alphabet by Lois Ehlert (Harcourt Brace and Company)

Vegan friends of ours gave us a copy of Wisconsin native Lois Ehlert's wonderful board book *Eating the Alphabet* years ago, and it's still a favorite. Lois Ehlert's Caldecott-winning children's books are alive with vibrant colors, and her collages are just beautiful. So many of her books are a natural part of every infant's library, and they traditionally share a shelf with Eric Carle's *Very Hungry Caterpillar.* The big, noticeable difference between Carle's gastronomic tome and Lois's *Eating the Alphabet* is that one book is vegan and the other—well, sorry caterpillar fans—is not.

The interesting thing about *Eating the Alphabet* that I think is worth pointing out is it doesn't have to be "vegan edited" like many other children's books. Lois Ehlert takes us from A to Z without once stopping at "C" is for chicken, "P" is for pork, or "W" is for water buffalo. To be specific, the author didn't use cheese or eggs.

This might be overlooked to some, but to me there is a very powerful message in this book that resonates every time I read it.

The Forgotten Rabbit by Nancy Furstinger (The Gryphon Press)
Known for her wonderful writing about animals and related issues, this charming book by Nancy Furstinger (and illustrated by Nancy Lane) follows rescued rabbit Bella on her journey from a neglected life in cruel conditions to a joy-filled home with someone who loves her. Both The Gryphon Press and Furstinger are active in raising awareness about animal issues, and the book includes a full page of information about rabbit adoption, proper bunny care, and other resources.

Jasper's Story: Saving Moon Bears by Jill Robinson (Sleeping Bear Press)
In this beautifully illustrated book, Jill Robinson (founder of the nonprofit Animals Asia) collaborates with renowned writer Marc Bekoff to tell the story of Jasper, one of the hundreds of bears rescued by Animals Asia from the cruelty of bear-bile farming. The book— illustrated by Gijsbert van Frankenhuyzen—offers an explanation of the bile-farming industry in simple terms, while depicting Jasper's inspiring recovery and happy new life at Animals Asia's sanctuary in China.

Lena of Vegitopia and the Mystery of the Missing Animals: A Vegan Fairy Tale by Sybil Severin (Vegan Publishers)
Lena of Vegitopia and the Mystery of the Missing Animals is a vegan-themed fairy tale about how one brave little girl stands up for the animal friends of her land and helps rescue them from being eaten. The book promotes messages of kindness, compassion, and action, and shows that magical things can happen when you harness the power of veggies.

Libby Finds Vegan Sanctuary by Julia Feliz Brueck (Vegan Publishers)

The first board book for little vegan readers! *Libby Finds Vegan Sanctuary* is the story of how a turkey inspires compassion and ultimately finds safety. Through colorful pages and a simple story fit for little hands, the board book helps young children understand the meaning of sanctuary and lightly explores the idea of choosing to prevent harm of other living beings. The story is based on a real-life rescued turkey, Libby, who lives in a farm animal sanctuary in Florida.

Make Way for Ducklings by Robert McCloskey (Puffin Books)

As mentioned, not all childhood classics will be appropriate for vegan households, but this beloved book (first published in 1941 and written and illustrated by Robert McCloskey) contains no scenes featuring animal cruelty. The story follows a pair of ducks as they search Boston for an appropriate home to begin their family. Finally finding just the right place, they are soon parents to eight baby birds. Escorting the little ones around town could be dangerous, but with the help of some compassionate humans, the ducks make their way to safety.

The One and Only Ivan by Katherine Applegate (HarperCollins)

This book is about a silverback gorilla named Ivan who lives in a cage at a mall. It is written in first person from the point of view of Ivan. In 2013, it was named the winner of the Newbery Medal.

Our Farm: By the Animals of Farm Sanctuary by Maya Gottfried (Knopf Books for Young Readers)

Maya Gottfried was inspired from her very first visit to a Farm Sanctuary. She realized that these places of peace provide loving shelter for animals who have suffered. *Our Farm: By the Animals of Farm Sanctuary* tells the stories of some of the residents of the organization's shelters in poems penned from the animals' perspectives. Art by Robert Rahway Zakanitch beautifully captures their sweet faces and gentle souls.

Piggy and Dad Go Fishing by David Martin (Scholastic)

In this book, a son sees the world in a completely different way, making emotional connections with animals, and shares his views with his dad. Piggy thinks the fish are sad, and in the end, they come up with a better form of "fishing"—which is feeding the fish rather than catching them. This teaches kids (and adults) that you can enjoy nature by being a part of it without taking from it or harming animals. I experienced a similar situation with my own kids—my oldest was interested in fishing, but we found a better way. In the heat of the summer, we visit dried-up creek beds and find fish who have been trapped in puddles and rescue them by moving them back to the water. If your child asks to go fishing, find other ways they can enjoy nature.

Rah, Rah, Radishes! and *Go, Go, Grapes!* by April Pulley Sayre (Little Simon)

Veggies take the stage in a rollicking ode to healthy eating in this classic board book edition of *Rah, Rah, Radishes!* We read this one at least three times a week to our kids. And, sweet fruits get their turn in *Go, Go, Grapes!*

Steven the Vegan by Dan Bodenstein (Totem Tales Publishing)

Steven and his classmates go on a field trip to a local farm sanctuary. While there, Steven's classmates learn that he is a vegan. Steven, along with many of the farm animals, teach his friends why, for him, animals are his friends, not his food. The idea of not eating meat or drinking milk may open a child up to ridicule and harassment, but *Steven the Vegan* gives these children ideas on how to deal with the situation and how to explain their beliefs. Each day, more children are being introduced to the concept of the vegan lifestyle.

'Twas the Night Before Thanksgiving by Dav Pilkey (Scholastic Paperbacks)

The incomparable Dav Pilkey adapts Clement Moore's classic Christmas poem to tell this wacky Thanksgiving tale. The day before Thanksgiving, eight boys and girls take a field trip to a turkey farm. They have fun playing with eight exuberant turkeys but are shocked to learn that Farmer Mack

Nuggett plans to kill all the turkeys for Thanksgiving dinners. So the children decide to smuggle all the turkeys home, and all their Thanksgiving dinners become vegetarian this year. The turkeys' lives are saved!

Waiting for Wings by Lois Ehlert (HMH Books for Young Readers; first edition)

Every spring, butterflies emerge and dazzle the world with their vibrant beauty. But where do butterflies come from? How are they born? What do they eat—and how?

With a simple rhyming text and glorious color-drenched collage, Lois Ehlert provides clear answers to these and other questions as she follows the life cycle of four common butterflies, from their beginnings as tiny hidden eggs and hungry caterpillars to their transformation into full-grown butterflies.

We're Vegan by Anna Bean (CreateSpace Independent Publishing Platform)

We're Vegan is the best children's book I've read about veganism since Ruby Roth's *Vegan is Love*. Bright, beautiful illustrations and the perfect amount of prose to inform and entertain touch on all the key points of being vegan.

I had an opportunity to talk with the author about her book and asked her what she wanted readers to get from it.

"I want readers to gain an understanding of what veganism is—that it is not merely a diet or a lifestyle, but a philosophy based on the values of compassion and justice, and it seeks to end *all* animal use," Anna says. "I want children (and adults too, of course) to understand that there is another way to live without relying on the use and abuse of animals. I've tried to explain this in a way that a small child can understand."

While I agree that the writing is perfect for small children, I really think it's also very fitting for grown adults. As an ethical vegan, I'm constantly asked the usual "why" and "how" questions, and Anna answers them in a very approachable and thoughtful way. This book is for everyone who has ever wondered what it means to be vegan.

Anna adds, "The book kind of just 'arrived' in my head one day! I've been a vegan for over thirty years but have only just started writing children's books. I will be releasing another one soon.

"Ever since I was a small child, I wanted to dedicate my life to helping animals. Eventually, I worked out that rather than being a vet (my initial career choice), the best way I could help animals is to be vegan and to promote veganism. I am so grateful that there are now many others who share this view and who are working together to end the use and abuse of animals by humans."

All proceeds from the sale of the book go toward feeding rescued animals.

When the World Is Dreaming by Rita Gray (HMH Books for Young Readers)

Children are big dreamers (and dreams directly follow bedtime stories!), so it's fitting that we have two children's books about dreams on this list. In lulling poetry, the book—written by Rita Gray and illustrated by Kenard Pak—asks what animals such as snakes, deer, and newts dream of. The end of the book will especially speak to young vegans, when a little girl dreams of all of the animals gathering in her room "and none of them feels the least bit afraid."

Yertle the Turtle by Dr. Seuss (Random House; First Edition edition)

There are lots great messages in this book about a greedy turtle who seeks to rule more and more of the world on the backs (literally) of less fortunate turtles. His plan doesn't work out, of course, and there is a wonderful quote that should send a great message to anyone reading it: "And the turtles, of course . . . all the turtles are FREE. As turtles, and maybe ALL creatures, should be."

Books to help vegan parents and parents-to-be:
- *The Kind Mama: A Simple Guide to Supercharged Fertility, a Radiant Pregnancy, a Sweeter Birth, and a Healthier, More Beautiful Beginning* by Alicia Silverstone (Rodale Books)

- *Raising Vegan Children in a Non-Vegan World: A Complete Guide for Parents* by Erin Pavlina (VegFamily.com)
- *Above All, Be Kind: Raising a Humane Child in Challenging Times* by Zoe Weil (New Society Publishers)
- *Help! There's a Vegan Coming for Dinner!* by Karen Jennings (Art and Soul Interiors)
- *The Vegan Pregnancy Survival Guide* by Sayward Rebhal (Herbivore Books)
- *Vegan for Her* by Virginia Messina and JL Fields (Da Capo Lifelong Books)
- *The Everything Vegan Pregnancy Book* by Reed Mangels (Everything)
- *Becoming Vegan* by Brenda Davis and Vesanto Melina (Book Pub Co.)
- *Skinny Bitch Bun in the Oven* by Rory Freedman and Kim Barnouin (Running Press)
- *Mind If I Order the Cheeseburger?* by Sherry F. Colb (Lantern Books)
- *The Skeptical Vegan* by Eric C. Lindstrom (Skyhorse Publishing)
- *Living the Farm Sanctuary Life* by Gene Baur (Rodale Books)
- *Plant-Powered Families* by Dreena Burton (BenBella Books)

Must-see films with a vegan message:

Charlotte's Web

Wilbur the pig is in danger of being slaughtered until his friend Charlotte the spider steps in to show everyone just how remarkable he really is! *Charlotte's Web* is a classic story that has inspired millions of people around the world to take a hint from Charlotte and take a closer look at the animals they consider to be "food."

Chicken Run

On a farm in England, chickens in a coop lay eggs day in and day out—and if they don't, they're the farmer's dinner. Ginger, the smartest chicken in the coop, wants everyone to escape! Then one day, a chicken named Rocky comes crash landing into the yard, and their luck changes.

Babe

One of the classic movies about animal rights, Babe is a heartwarming tale of a pig who proves that he's worth more than just ending up as a holiday meal. Taken from his mother on a factory farm when he is only a tiny piglet, Babe is adopted into a family of dogs who are used to herd sheep on a farm. A friend to all, Babe shows everyone on the farm just how smart and sweet pigs can be when they're only given the chance.

Bee Movie

Bee Movie touches primarily on topics of exploitation and of animals living a life of slavery. In one scene, Barry the bee exclaims, "Is this what nature intended for us? To be forcibly addicted to smoke machines and man-made wooden slat work camps? Living out our lives as honey slaves to the white man?" In another scene, Barry finds an ally in a cow who, in relating to his plight, cries, "Milk, cream, cheese; it's all me. And I don't see a nickel! Sometimes I just feel like a piece of meat!" Lines like this may leave children wondering whether bees and cows actually "give" humans their honey and milk or whether their secretions are taken from them as part of an unjust exploitation process.

Bambi

Follow Bambi, a curious young deer, as he and his friends Thumper the rabbit, Flower the skunk, and the wise Friend Owl play together and frolic in the woods that they call home. This classic animated tale will teach you lessons about love, life, and the evils of hunting.

Dumbo

Dumbo and his mother are forced to perform in the circus, until his mother goes crazy from the stress and is separated from her baby and locked up. Alone and heartbroken, Dumbo is miserable in circus life and desperate to be seen as the special little elephant he really is. This film will really resonate with children, with Ringling Brothers Circus now a thing of the past.

E.T. the Extra-Terrestrial

After a gentle alien is stranded on Earth, it is discovered and befriended by a young boy named Elliott (Henry Thomas). Bringing the extra-terrestrial into his suburban California house, Elliott introduces E.T., as the alien is dubbed, to his brother and his little sister, Gertie (Drew Barrymore), and the children decide to keep its existence a secret.

Ferdinand

In a partnership between the animal sanctuary The Gentle Barn and the major film production company Twentieth Century Fox, the end of 2017 saw the release of *Ferdinand*, a film about misunderstood animals and their right to be free. This animated film was promoted heavily in the vegan community as having a very powerful animal rights message and is great for all PG-rated audience members.

Finding Nemo (and Finding Dory)

Fish belong in the ocean, not in a tank or on anyone's plate! Nemo is "fish-napped" from his friends and family by divers who want to stick him in a tank on display. His dad goes on an epic adventure to save him, showing that fish feel pain, want to be free, and love their families—just like all other animals. It even includes one of our favorite slogans: "Fish are friends, not food!"

Free Willy

When maladjusted orphan Jesse (Jason James Richter) vandalizes a theme park, he is placed with foster parents and must work at the park to make amends. There, he meets Willy, a young orca whale who has been separated from his family. Sensing kinship, they form a bond and, with the help of kindly whale trainer Rae Lindley (Lori Petty), develop a routine of tricks. However, greedy park owner Dial (Michael Ironside) soon catches wind of the duo and makes plans to profit from them.

Pete's Dragon

Mr. Meacham (Robert Redford), a woodcarver, delights local children with stories of a mysterious dragon that lives deep in the woods of the

Pacific Northwest. His daughter Grace (Bryce Dallas Howard) believes these are just tall tales, until she meets Pete (Oakes Fegley), a ten-year-old orphan who says he lives in the woods with a giant, friendly dragon. With help from a young girl named Natalie (Oona Laurence), Grace sets out to investigate if this fantastic claim is true.

Online resources:

There are countless excellent Facebook groups you can join as a vegan parent. Simply search for them in the Facebook search box, choose "groups," and either join or request to join. Browse the pages and post any questions you might have. In fact, when writing this book, I crowdsourced some of these lists and ideas from other vegan parents. We all want to help each other and help the animals, and I'm confident you will find a supportive online community.

Search "vegan recipes" on Pinterest and Instagram for even more inspiration for amazing snacks and meals for your vegan kids. Be sure to check out one of my favorite Instagram accounts, @kaylees_vegan_lunchbox, for bright and colorful lunchbox ideas.

Here are other websites of interest:

EasyVegetarian.net: Thinking of becoming vegetarian/vegan, want to understand why a family member or friend is VEGetariAN, or want to understand the basics of VEGetariANism and its implications for animals, humans, and the environment? Visit this resource.

GirlieGirlArmy: According to their website, "GirlieGirl Army is your Glamazon Guide to Green Living, a one-stop online resource for a ferociously progressive, urban-minded approach to cruelty-free living. We don't carry picket signs; we carry designer clutches. We don't preach; we polish. Our message is simple: You can live large and still make a positive impact. You can be eco-conscious and elegant."

PetaKids.com: So much fun! It's super easy to help animals, no matter how old you are. Learn all about why you should help animals used for food, clothing, entertainment, and experimentation, plus how to protect companion animals and wildlife!

RaiseVegan.com: All around an excellent source of information for vegan parents. The goal of Vegan Pregnancy and Parenting, the Facebook group that is managed by RaiseVegan, is to provide caring education and support to vegans and to people who want to become vegan. Their belief in living a peaceful life is never-ending and is always striving for improvement.

VeganKidsMagazine.com: This Australian magazine brings together inspiring vegans, vegan health professionals, vegan families, and, of course, vegan kids to educate and inspire each other on the vegan message.

TheVeganMom.com: Award-winning vegan blog by Lisa, a vegan mom who offers ideas for other vegan moms, lists resources for vegan parents, and offers a list of family-friendly cookbooks.

VegYouth.com: Meet Chloe, the founder of Vegetarian and Vegan Youth. She started VegYouth in August 2013 when she was sixteen years old and in the eleventh grade. Five years later, she's still as passionate about veganism.

YoungVeggie.org: From the Vegetarian Society, a not-for-profit in the United Kingdom, this site provides insight on being vegan and being British. It's very informative to see the different messaging and products the Brits recommend for easy vegan living.

Vegan activities and road trips for your little activists:
Visit an actual animal sanctuary

There are amazing sanctuaries all over the country where families can visit and learn about the lives of farm animals, including Farm Sanctuary and Woodstock Sanctuary (both of which happen to be near me in New York). While you're there, take a tour, pet the rescues, and hear their stories of salvation. This should be on your to-do list once your kids turn five, and return once a year to say "hi" to old friends and meet the new rescues.

Gene Baur is the cofounder and president of Farm Sanctuary. In the 1980s, after traveling around the United States and learning about agriculture, Baur began investigations into factory farms, stockyards, and slaughterhouses. He believed the conditions he observed were unacceptable, and these experiences helped motivate the creation of Farm Sanctuary, which created the sanctuary movement in North America. He is also the author of two best-selling books, *Farm Sanctuary: Changing Hearts and Minds About Animals and Food* and *Living the Farm Sanctuary Life: The Ultimate Guide to Eating Mindfully, Living Longer, and Feeling Better Every Day*. Gene knows a thing or two about the importance of the farm sanctuary experience for all ages.

"At Farm Sanctuary, cows, pigs, chickens, and other farm animals are our friends, not our food," Gene tells me. "They were rescued from slaughter, and upon arriving at the sanctuary, they are able to experience human kindness for the first time. It is wonderful to see the animals' lives transformed as they finally feel safe and are able to heal.

"On modern 'farms,' animals are confined by the thousands in warehouses where they are seen as unfeeling production units. Millions are confined in cages and crates so tightly that they can barely move, and they routinely endure painful mutilations like castration, de-beaking, and tail docking without painkillers. The conditions are so severe that hundreds of millions of farm animals die every year before reaching the slaughterhouse. Their deaths are callously calculated as acceptable economic losses.

"Most consumers don't think very much about the way we eat, but food represents one of our most intimate connections with earth and defines our relationships with other animals. How we treat other animals says a lot about us. If Mahatma Gandhi was correct when he famously said, 'You can judge the moral progress of a nation by its treatment of animals,' we have much to atone for. Exploiting and killing animals for food affects our physical and psychological well-being, and disregarding their suffering undermines our ability to act with compassion. Violence creates more violence, and it can easily jump the species barrier.

"Abusing animals requires that we lose part of our empathy, which is a very important part of our humanity. This also can lead us to disparage and demean our victims in order to rationalize and validate our abusive conduct. We belittle those we harm and try to convince ourselves that they don't know or deserve better. It is not a compliment in our society, for example, to be called a 'pig' or a 'turkey.'

"While consumers may not think very much about the animals who are exploited for food, we are responsible for their suffering if we eat meat, milk, and eggs. Slaughterhouses and factory farms only exist because people buy their products. The good news is that we can live well without consuming animal foods, and each of us can make a positive difference by eating plants instead."

Visiting a local farm sanctuary is the ideal way to help your young one make the connection.

Volunteer at your local SPCA

All animal shelters are full of animals in need of love and attention. Visit your local animal shelter and walk a dog or pet a cat. This is a rewarding activity as long as you're prepared to hear and respond to, "Can we bring him home?" every fifteen minutes. Ask the shelter if you can make or bring anything to help with the animals.

Plant an actual garden

Whether you have a vast field or a couple of pots on a windowsill, plant some herbs or your favorite veggies. When it's time to harvest, delight in preparing homecooked meals with your bounty (recipes in this book, page 168, and online). Kids love to see seeds become plants and especially love the idea of grabbing a tomato or cucumber right off the vine and taking a bite.

Make a backyard bird/animal feeder

Create a squirrel, butterfly, or bird feeder, and rejoice in visits from animal friends all year long. The best way to keep squirrels from attacking your bird feeder? Feed them from their own feeder. You can Google "squirrel feeder" for some pretty creative ideas.

Visit a working fruit or vegetable farm

Call ahead and take a trip to a nearby vegetable or fruit farm. Find out if they have events and opportunities for you to help out while you are visiting. Many will also allow self-picking, which is truly the best way to teach your little vegan "where food comes from."

Take a hike (literally)

Visit a wildlife preserve, waterfall, hiking trail, mountain climb, or an extra-large backyard, and take in the nature and animals around you. Be sure to observe. As the saying goes, "Take nothing but pictures. Leave nothing but footprints. Kill nothing but time." While exploring this incredible planet, keep a logbook of the plants and animals you find and research them online when you get home.

Shop at a farmer's market

Check your local area for the schedule of your farmer's market and also see if they have any indoor markets during the off-season. Take a trip and pick up fresh produce. Talk about what you're buying (and sample along the way). Then, take your bounty home and plan a meal.

Go bird-watching

With the thousands of species among the various regions of the world, this activity offers unlimited opportunities for creating an enriching animal experience. Bring a notepad, a birder guide, and some binoculars, and get the kids outdoors to explore.

Camp at a national park

Plan a day trip or overnight outing at one of the thousands of national parks in the United States, and observe animals in their natural habitats (from a safe distance). I've spent hundreds of hours camping, and there is no better way to get to know just how wild wildlife can be—especially when you're sleeping on the ground.

Visit a fruit or vegetable festival

Do some online research for a list of seasonal festivals in your area. These events typically offer food, activities, and entertainment for the whole family, and many are based on harvest/local produce. Sadly, some are also focused on meat; avoid those.

Take a vegan cooking class

This fun activity gets the whole family in the kitchen, improves everyone's skills, and introduces the family to new recipes. Check with your local co-op or grocery store to see if they have any upcoming vegan cooking events—or ask if you can host one yourself.

Table at a VegFest or animal rights event

Groups like PETA, Farm Animal Rights Movement, Mercy for Animals, and more are often looking for volunteers to help hand out literature or manage their table at VegFests and other animal rights events. Sign yourself up for a shift and bring your kids along. They will meet other vegan kids as well as learn more about the horrors of animal agriculture.

Get involved in a demonstration or protest

Like the tabling idea, these same vegan and animal rights groups conduct demonstrations and protests nearly every weekend and some weeknights. They are always looking for more hands to help hold signs and increase exposure for their messaging. Email their grassroots manager and ask to be informed when the next event takes place near you.

Host and attend vegan potlucks

Ah, the backbone of veganism: the potluck. Invite vegan and non-vegan friends to show off their creative cooking skills, and make a theme for the potluck (chili cook-off, mac and cheese, etc.). Kids love these events, and there is always something they'll love to eat. Since making my own life-changing, lane-changing, game-changing shift in thinking, some of my more popular potluck dishes include:

Pizza: Homemade, gluten-free, and vegan, and every bit as good as a meat and dairy cheese pizza. In fact, you can top it with some pretty convincing alt-meats (like a ground beef or shredded chick'n). The kids will love it.

Soy chorizo: I originally discovered the soy chorizo at Trader Joe's but have since made my own homemade version (using TVP)—and it's pretty amazing. Somewhat spicy but delicious, and perfect in tacos.

Macaroni and cheese: Some soy milk, a little vegan butter, and dairy-free cheese (and maybe some nutritional yeast to boost up the B12). Melt all that over a low burner and pour over gluten-free elbow macaroni. You can broil it at the end to get that crispy top, if you prefer.

Chocolate chunk cookies: Remember that episode of *Friends* when Monica was trying to duplicate Phoebe's incredible chocolate chip cookie recipe, and it turned out the recipe was printed on the bag of chocolate chips? Well, like anything you've done in the past, that recipe works the same—just use vegan ingredients.

Burritos and tacos: Pretty much all variations of Mexican cuisine translate beautifully to vegan and travel well to potlucks. Don't forget the vegan sour cream.

Lasagna: Red or white, this layered pasta dish is the perfect addition to any potluck, and it'll go fast. This is the case with most casserole dishes. Bring plenty.

Broccoli quiche: Perfect for any brunch. Completely egg- and dairy-free when you use Follow Your Heart's vegan egg and their incredible smoked gouda.

Fettuccine Alfredo: There is so much you can do with cashews, and this Alfredo sauce rivals any out there. Cashews also make wonderful creams.

Sweet potato fries: Toss cut sweet potato in sesame oil, garlic powder, and paprika and bake at 400 degrees for 30 minutes (flip once midway). Serve with chipotle Vegenaise dipping sauce. Shut the front door.

Pão de queijo: Simple and gluten-free Brazilian cheese bread, or pão de queijo, made with tapioca flour and dairy-free cheese. Seriously, kids will kill each other for this, bringing new meaning to "the Hunger Games." **Pro tip:** there is a boxed version of this from Chebe.

Salads: Yes, I eat salads, too. Probably not as many as I should, but I also cut myself some slack here, since eating all these other foods is so much fun! Note: both potato and macaroni salads are simple to veganize.

There you have it! You're now a vegan pro. Walk into that birthday party, holiday event, school PTO meeting, or potluck, with your vegan kids in tow and your head held high. You've done it. You're now the proud parent of a vegan kid.

You go, vegan.

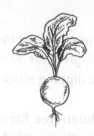

EPILOGUE

"Man begets, but land does not beget."
—*Cecil Rhodes*

Well, look at you. You're almost done reading this book, and now your confidence level about raising vegan kids is through the roof.

They're not going to shrivel away from a lack of nutrition. They won't die of protein-deficiency. They won't become prey to life's predators. They *will* become the cool kid in their classroom that other kids talk about to their parents when they get home. It's not only possible to raise kids vegan—it's optimal.

Optimal for their health, the health of the earth, and the health and well-being of billions of animals with whom we share this planet.

Whether you're doing it for your kids for health reasons, for the environment, or for the animals, veganism is about to explode world-wide, and getting your whole family on board now is part of this turning tide.

The best time to go vegan is always now.

Many other parents have successfully raised vegan kids, and now you're armed with the information to do it yourself. Share this book (or, better yet, buy someone their own copy). Every parent or parent-to-be should read this to understand the importance of raising healthy and compassionate kids.

And every parent should start today.

As long as we're breeding, we may as well be breeding vegans—right? The future of humankind counts on us to usher in future generations as vegans: hundreds, thousands, and millions of us.

We can become a vegan army. This is our Kale of Duty. Vegans *will* win this war, through peaceful means (and veggie burgers).

We not only have the largest land animals on our side in this war—behemoths like elephants, rhinos, gorillas, and bison (all vegan) —we also have powerhouse bodybuilders like Robert Cheeke, Torre Washington, and Amanda Riester (all vegan); we have an ever-growing list of elite athletes like David Carter, John Salley, and Tia Blanco (all vegan); and to keep the troops entertained, we have celebrities like Joaquin Phoenix, Woody Harrelson, and Carrie Underwood, just to name a few.

Big Agriculture is getting desperate. They are waging their *own* war to keep their myths alive and promote meat, dairy, and eggs to consumers who, in turn, feed these dangerous foods to their young. They are backed by lobbying groups and massive budgets. They will do what it takes to dig their heels in to protect their investments. It's a vicious cycle that has to end.

And it all starts with you. Today.

As nondairy milks and meatless meats soar in popularity, Big Ag is trying to squash plant-based sales and even cheat consumers. Compassion Over Killing, a Washington, DC–based animal rights group, helped form a class action suit against 70 percent of the dairy industry for raising prices by slaughtering five hundred thousand young cows (consumers are now owed a $52 million settlement), and a similar suit has been filed against major US chicken producers. As dairy sales drop because of healthier plant-based options, Big Dairy is also looking to the Food and Drug Administration (FDA) to block the use of words like "milk" and "cheese" on dairy-free product labels—a sure sign of desperate times calling for desperate measures.

A bipartisan group of thirty-two members of Congress is asking the FDA to crack down on companies that call plant-based beverages "milk," saying that FDA regulations define milk as a "lacteal secretion."

Mmmm. Got Lacteal Secretion? When you put it that way, "nut milk" sounds downright delicious.

The European Union (EU) Court of Justice confirmed a ban on products of a "purely plant-based substance" using words like milk, cream, butter, cheese, or yogurt in their marketing—terms reserved by EU law for milk of animal origin or products directly derived from cow's milk. (Except for coconut milk; for some reason, they can look the other way when it comes to coconuts.)

Major brands are seeing the potential of vegan eats as well. ConAgra acquired LightLife, manufacturers of plant-based foods; and Daiya, arguably the first mainstream vegan cheese company, was bought out by Japanese pharmaceutical company Otsuka for $325.97 million. Investors from every industry, like Bill Gates and Biz Stone, and even celebrities like Leonardo DiCaprio, are investing millions of dollars into the alt-meat market.

If you can't beat them, join them, right? Tyson, the largest meat producer in the United States, has invested in plant-based meat company Beyond Meat. Major chains are offering vegan options because consumers are asking for them, from Subway to Dunkin' Donuts and Starbucks (complete list starting on page 142). Taco Bell and Chipotle even released easy guides to ordering their popular vegan options, and fast food chains not getting on the vegan bandwagon are getting left behind. McDonald's is closing hundreds of locations due to decreased sales brought on by more intelligent, health-conscious consumers (but is now test marketing the McVegan burger as a way to compete).

The alt-meat industry has expanded so much over the last year that my most recent book, *The Skeptical Vegan*, is already outdated (it came out just a year ago in 2017). Vegan options are both amazing-tasting and readily available. Beyond Meat has introduced the Beyond Burger and started selling this amazing product in *meat aisles* across the United States (as well as test-marketing them in various TGIFriday's locations). The Herbivorous Butcher, a Minneapolis-based vegan butcher, was named reader's choice in *USA Today*'s "Best Food & Drink Maker" in the *nation* in a poll against nonvegan competitors. Major publications spotlighted vegan foods, and Nathaniel Johnson from *Grist* said: "Someday, we'll look back at 2016 as the year we realized we might be perfectly happy to give up meat."

And that's just the beginning. Plant-based is expected to be a top global food trend in the coming years, and 2018 is expected to usher in even more changes toward a more sustainable, vegan, future. The link between animal products and climate change is clear, and young people are becoming more aware of their responsibility in turning back the clock on the damage already done.

The science is clear. Animal agriculture is a leading cause of environmental devastation, from deforestation to ocean dead zones to air pollution. One recent study published in *PNAS* showed that if the whole world went vegan, food-related greenhouse gas emissions would be cut by 70 percent and 8 million human lives would be saved by 2050. The United Nations published a 2009 report that says, "A substantial reduction of impacts [from agriculture] would only be possible with a substantial worldwide diet change away from animal products." In other words, vegan eating could save the planet.

Additionally, the public is finally standing up and saying no to animals in entertainment.

After years of slowing sales and declining attendance, Ringling Bros. and Barnum & Bailey Circus announced in 2017 that it is permanently closing after more than 140 years in business. Even the biggest name in animal "entertainment" cited declining attendance and changing public views about using performing animals. Next to go? SeaWorld. Films like 2013's *Blackfish* shed a powerful light on the lives of orcas and other captive marine life, and, one by one, tanks are being emptied and breeding has already been stopped at most aquariums around the country.

Healthcare pros tout the benefits of plant-based eating in bestselling books and dynamic documentary films, suitable even for the youngest vegans.

"They will get more of the good stuff and less of the bad," says Dr. Barnard, who was featured in the documentaries *Super Size Me*, *Forks Over Knives*, and *What the Health*. "Children who follow vegetarian diets, especially vegan diets, are at a reduced risk for being overweight or obese, compared with children who follow nonvegetarian diets. And of course, a healthy weight in childhood increases the likelihood of not being overweight or obese as adults. They also consume more fruits and vegetables, fewer sweets and salty snacks, and less fat and saturated fat.

"And plant-based foods are the ones your child should have as he or she starts consuming food other than breast milk (or formula). Exposing children to healthful foods right from the start sets them up for having healthier preferences for the long run."

Further proving that the health power of a plant-based diet has made it into the public consciousness now more than ever, many medical doctors now acknowledge that a healthy vegan diet can prevent (or even reverse) heart disease, types of cancer, obesity, type 2 diabetes, and other chronic ailments. Kaiser Permanente recommends plant-based eating; Physicians Committee for Responsible Medicine (PCRM) opened the vegan-focused Barnard Medical Center in the nation's capital, and events like International Plant-Based Nutrition Healthcare Conference and Remedy Food Project are growing rapidly and attracting thousands of people from around the country to think about what they're eating.

Plus, people worldwide are more interested in veganism than ever.

Search queries on Google show a major rise in vegan search terms, including "vegan food nearby" and "going vegan" over the past three years, with a huge spike at the end of 2016. From Australia to Italy to Germany, people all over the world are more interested in a plant-based lifestyle than ever before.

Google itself is touting plant-based foods, and their CEO Eric Schmidt has committed to a more vegan future for the company and sees this as the trend for the world. Schmidt, who is also executive chairman of Google's parent company, Alphabet, predicts that a plant-based revolution is coming. "Replacing livestock with growing and harvesting plants will reduce greenhouse gas emissions and fight climate change," he stated. "The meat industry, particularly cattle producers, emit significant greenhouse gases."

Schmidt named the number one "game-changing" trend of the future as the consumption of plant-based proteins instead of meat. He added that alt-meats will become the standard over time.

~

Now, I recognize that we have a long road ahead of us with our own two little vegans. There are going to be obstacles and challenges along the way in keeping them on track. We will deal with each hurdle one at a time and remain optimistic. We've made this decision for them, as much as we've made this decision for us (and the animals). We want to wake up every morning, with our total four hours of sleep, knowing that we're no longer contributing to the cycle of confinement, abuse, and slaughter. We'll wake our babies up each day—oh, who am I kidding? They're up at 5:30 a.m. no matter what—knowing we've given them the tools to be healthy, compassionate humans.

There are more than 360,000 babies born each day worldwide. That's a potential 131,400,000 mouths to feed in just the next year. The current food system is neither healthy nor sustainable, but we have a choice now that will help the planet and future generations: going vegan.

Your life is your message to the world. Make sure it's inspiring.

One person can make a difference. Imagine what a difference your whole family will make. Change grows exponentially. The choice you make for yourself and your family will have a direct effect on others and their families. One by one, we will *all* make a difference.

Go vegan.

ACKNOWLEDGMENTS

"Gratitude is the memory of the heart."

—*Anonymous*

Thanks always go straight to Skyhorse Publishing and my editor, Kim Lim, for being at my beck and call with the numerous email questions all year long and for spotting, and fixing, all my errors and making me look so good. The fact that she actually found me and asked me to write *The Skeptical Vegan* will always be one of the major turning points of my life. One day (soon), I will make the trip to New York City and take her out for breakfast at Champ's Diner, then lunch at the Cinnamon Snail, and dinner at Hangawi. I hope she's hungry for some of the best vegan food in the country.

I'd also like to thank my wife, Jen, for encouraging us to have not one, but two, vegan babies. It's because of her beauty and constant support that they, and this book, exist. I'll always say that Paisley and Cooper will keep me young, because at this point, considering their energy levels, I won't live to be fifty-five.

They are exhausting. Ask anyone who knows them. Vegan baby power.

I *need* to thank my own mom, Peg. While she didn't raise me and my two sisters vegan (far from it), she did raise the three of us as a single mom on a meager salary, and we never wanted for anything. She kept us safe, happy, and fed. She taught me how to be grateful, and I'm not sure she even realizes this. For this, I am forever thankful.

Thank you to all the vegans who have embraced me and supported me since I started my journey, and thank you to everyone, and hopefully soon-to-be vegans, for reading *The Skeptical Vegan*. Every time I read a positive review, it truly makes me feel blessed. And whenever I read a bad review, I am equally grateful that someone took the time to tell me how they feel. No one ever learns from successes; we learn from life's failures and setbacks, and we improve upon ourselves from there.

Speaking of learning from setbacks, I think about how I spent the first half my life *not* vegan. They say that the only regret vegans have is that they didn't go vegan sooner. You have this unique opportunity to make sure you, your offspring, and maybe *their* offspring, are vegan. For life.

If someone told me ten years ago that I would have written two books about going vegan, I never, in a million years, would have believed them. That was the furthest thought in my mind back then, but today, I am proud that veganism has become my entire identity.

Thank you to all the amazing contributors to this book. You are the glue that holds together my own experiences, stories, and anecdotes. You have added an incredible amount of wisdom, practical advice, and insight into vegan parenting that I am sure countless others will learn from. I'm confident your words will make a difference for hundreds of parents and their littles.

Words that will also make a difference for the animals.

Thank you all.

Special thank you to:

Keith Allison

Dr. Neal Barnard

Shannon Blair

Dr. Tom Campbell

Jessica Carlson

Maura Cummings

Christine Day

Sarvar Dhillon

Michael Dorf

Robin Fetter

Benjamin Finegan

JL Fields

Cindy Ford

Lewis Freedman

Daisy Fuentes

J.D. Goldschmidt

Steve Glover
Colleen Patrick-Goudreau
Amie Hamlin
Emily Harlan
Alex Hershaft
Kevin Hicks
Sarah Johnson-Dwyer
Satish Karandikar
Gillian Lindstrom
Peg Lindstrom
Kristina Parker
Claire Lunny-Peters
Jennifer Majka
Richard Marx
Jenny Miller
Matthew Modine

Robin Molito-Moore
Themistoklis Monachos
Victoria Moran
Kristina Parker
Brian Patton
Jen Riley
Ryan Ritchie
Craig Robinson
Ari Salomon
Allison Rivers Samson
Nathan Runkle
Heather Swift
Skyhorse Publishing
Vegan Babies
VegNews Magazine
Jason Wrobel

Contributors:

- Keith Allison, *field educator, Ethical Choices Program*
- Dr. Neal Barnard, *nutrition researcher, bestselling author, and one of America's leading advocates for health, nutrition, and higher standards in research*
- Shannon Blair, *mother of PETA's 2017 Cutest Kid: Evan the Vegan*
- Gene Baur, *Farm Sanctuary founder and president, and author of* Living the Farm Sanctuary Life
- Dr. Tom Campbell, MD, *author of* The China Study Solution, *co-author of* The China Study, *and plant-based medical doctor*
- Robin Fetter, *CEO and Founder of VegParents Network and The Real Vegan Housewife*
- JL Fields, *culinary instructor and cookbook author of* The Vegan Air Fryer: The Healthier Way to Enjoy Deep-Fried Flavors
- Cindy Ford, *blogger at Silly Little Vegan and HappyCow Ambassador, Columbus, Ohio region*

- J.D. Goldschmidt, *vegan actor/model/personal trainer living in New York City*
- Colleen Patrick-Goudreau, *author,* The 30-Day Vegan Challenge
- Amie Hamlin, *executive director, The Coalition for Healthy School Food*
- Alex Hershaft, *founding president of Farm Animal Rights Movement (FARM)*
- Claire Lunny-Peters, *vegan chef, parent, and YouTube personality*
- Robin Molito-Moore, *humane educator, founder of RaisingVegKids.com and NYC Vegetarian and Vegan Families Meetup*
- Lorena Mucke, *founder and CEO of Ethical Choices Program*
- Kristina Parker, *vegan mom (Portland, OR)*
- Nathan Runkle, *founder and executive director of Mercy For Animals*
- Allison Rivers Samson, *award-winning author of* Veganize It! *and co-founder of Dairy Detox*

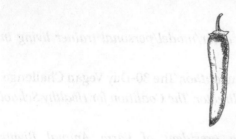

NOTES

CHAPTER 1 In the Beginning: Babies, Bottles, and Breasts

Pg. 3. "Cow's milk: When and how to introduce it," BabyCenter, LLC, last updated October 2016, https://www.babycenter.com/0_cows-milk-when-and-how-to-introduce-it_1334703.bc.

CHAPTER 2 Milk: It Does a Body Bad

Pg. 8. Erica M. Schulte, Nicole M. Avena, Ashley N. Gearhardt, "Which Foods May Be Addictive? The Roles of Processing, Fat Content, and Glycemic Load," *PLOS One* (Feb 2015), doi: 10.1371/journal.pone.0117959.

Pg. 9. Dr. T. Colin Campbell, *The China Study* (Dallas: BenBella Books, 2006).

Pg. 11. Karl Michaëlsson, Alicja Wolk, Sophie Langenskiöld, Samar Basu, Eva Warensjö Lemming, Håkan Melhus, Liisa Byberg, "Milk intake and risk of mortality and fractures in women and men: cohort studies," *British Medical Journal* (October 2014), doi: https://doi.org/10.1136/bmj.g6015.

Pg. 12. "Over 100 complaints received by ASAI over ad for 'plant-based' dairy milk," *The Journal*, November 14 2017, http://www.thejournal.ie/complaints-national-diary-council-plant-based-milk-ad-3696831-Nov2017/.

Pg. 12. Tami J. Cline, PhD, RD, SNS, "Fluid Milk in School Meal Programs," (National Dairy Council Study, 2015), https://www.milkmeansmore.org/wp-content/uploads/2016/05/DMI-Fluid-Milk-in-School-Meal-Programs.pdf.

Pg. 12. "Calcium: What's Best for Your Bones and Health?" (Harvard University School of Public Health, 2015), https://www.hsph.harvard.edu/nutritionsource/calcium-full-story/.

Pg. 15. Dr. Michael Greger, "Childhood Constipation & Cow's Milk," https://nutritionfacts.org/video/childhood-constipation-and-cows-milk/.

CHAPTER 3 Born Compassionate: Bite an Apple/Pet a Bunny

Pg. 18. Mark Hawthorne, "U.S. Prisons to Begin Offering Vegan Entrées in October 2016," (Striking at the Roots, 2016), https://strikingattheroots.wordpress.com/2016/09/22/u-s-prisons-to-begin-offering-vegan-entrees-in-october-2016/.

Pg. 28. Kate Stewart and Matthew Cole, "The Conceptual Separation of Food and Animals in Childhood" *Food, Culture and Society* (December 2009), https://doi.org/10.2752/175174409X456746.

Pg. 32. "Vegetarian Cats and Dogs," PETA, 2000, https://www.peta.org/living/animal-companions/vegetarian-cats-dogs/.

Pg. 32. "All About BSE (Mad Cow Disease)," U.S. Food & Drug Administration, last updated December 22, 2017, https://www.fda.gov/AnimalVeterinary/Resourcesfor You/AnimalHealthLiteracy/ucm136222.htm.

CHAPTER 4 Relearning the Food Pyramid: Turn Your Dinner Table Over

Pg. 36. "Flemish Institute of Health Life Guidelines," Flemish Institute of Healthy Living, 2017, https://www.gezondleven.be/themas/voeding/voedingsdriehoek.

Pg. 37. The International Agency for Research on Cancer (IARC), "Carcinogenicity of consumption of red and processed meat," *The Lancet Oncology* (October 2015), http://www.thelancet.com/journals/lanonc/article/PIIS1470-2045(15)00444-1/abstract.

Pg. 37. Shan-shan Wang, Sovichea Lay, Hai-ning Yu, and Sheng-rong Shen, "Dietary Guidelines for Chinese Residents (2016): comments and comparisons," *PubMed Central* (September 2016), doi: 10.1631/jzus.B1600341.

Pg. 41. "DDT is good for me-e-e! (1947)" Click Americana, accessed March 3, 2018, https://clickamericana.com/media/advertisements /ddt-is-good-for-me-e-e-1947.

CHAPTER 5 Veganizing Your Holidays: Santa Ain't Vegan, Bunnies Don't Lay Eggs, and the Halloween Switch Witch
Pg. 50. Shel Silverstein, *Where the Sidewalk Ends* (HarperCollins, 2014).

CHAPTER 7 The Doctor Is In: Your Family's Clean Bill of Health
Pg. 68. Christopher Duggan, John Watkins, W. Allan Walker, *Nutrition In Pediatrics* (Connecticut: PMPH-USA, 2008).

CHAPTER 8 A Shot in the Arm: Vaccinations and Herd Immunity
Pg. 79. Leah Zerbe, "10 Foods That Fight Cold and Flu," Rodale Wellness, published October 28, 2016, https://www.rodalewellness.com /living-well/cold-flu-remedies%3Fslide%3D1.
Pg. 79. N. Kumar, A. Banik, P. K. Sharma, "Use of Secondary Metabolite in Tuberculosis: A Review," *Der Pharma Chemica* (2010), http:// www.derpharmachemica.com/pharma-chemica/use-of -secondary-metabolite-in-tuberculosis-a-review.pdf.

CHAPTER 11 Animals Are Not Food: We Don't Eat Our Friends
Pg. 100. Richard Watts, *Vegan Sidekick*, Instagram, https:// www.instagram.com/vegansidekick.

CHAPTER 12 Lunch Lady Land: Hold the Steamed Cheeseburger
Pg. 114. Giuseppe Iacono, MD, Francesca Cavataio, MD, Giuseppe Montalto, MD, Ada Florena, MD, Mario Tumminello, MD, Maurizio Soresi, MD, Alberto Notarbartolo, MD, Antonio Carroccio, MD, "Intolerance of Cow's Milk and Chronic Constipation in Children," *New England Journal of Medicine* (October 1998), doi: 10.1056 /NEJM199810153391602.
Pg. 119. "Our Program," Ethical Choices Program, accessed March 5, 2018, http://www.ethicalchoicesprogram.org/our-program.

Pg. 122. Melia Robinson, "Generation Z is creating a $5 billion market for fake meat and seafood," Business Insider, published November 1, 2017, http://www.businessinsider.com/generation-z-is-eating-fake-meat-2017-10.

CHAPTER 15 Where to Turn: Getting Support

Pg. 150. "Ranking the Most (and Least) Vegetarian-Friendly Cities," *Priceonomics*, October 12, 2016, https://priceonomics.com/ranking-the-most-and-least-vegetarian-friendly/.

CHAPTER 16 My Parenting Mantra: Safe, Happy, and Fed

Pg. 159. "Top Trends in Prepared Foods 2017: Exploring trends in meat, fish and seafood; pasta, noodles and rice; prepared meals; savory deli food; soup; and meat substitutes," Report Buyer, June 2017, https://www.reportbuyer.com/product/4959853/.

Pg. 159. Ruth Brown, "Parents killed baby with quinoa 'milk' diet: authorities," *New York Post*, May 18, 2017, https://nypost.com/2017/05/18/parents-killed-baby-with-quinoa-milk-diet-authorities/.

CHAPTER 17 Eating All the Veggies (and More): Recipes for the Little Vegans

Pg. 161. "The meaning and origin of the expression: You are what you eat," The Phrase Finder, https://www.phrases.org.uk/meanings/you-are-what-you-eat.html.

EPILOGUE

Pg. 210. "The Herbivorous Butcher Named Best Food & Drink Maker in the USA!" *USA Today 10BEST*, accessed March 5, 2018, http://www.10best.com/awards/travel/makers-in-the-usa-best-food-drink-2016/.

Pg. 211. Nathaniel Johnson, "Guilty of Hamburglary" Grist.com, December 28, 2016, https://grist.org/briefly/the-vegan-meat-market-really-beefed-up-in-2016/.

Pg. 211. Marco Springmann, H. Charles J. Godfray, Mike Rayner, and Peter Scarborough, "Analysis and valuation of the health and climate change cobenefits of dietary change," *PNAS* (March 2016), https://doi.org/10.1073/pnas.1523119113.

Pg. 211. "The Lazy Person's Guide to Saving the World," United Nations, accessed March 5, 2018, http://www.un.org /sustainabledevelopment/takeaction/.

Pg. 212. Google Trends "vegan" search, Google Trends Data, 2016–2017, https://trends.google.com/trends/explore?q=vegan.

Pg. 212. Lauren Willis, "Google's Executive Chairman Predicts 'Vegan Revolution is Coming,'" Live Kindly, published September 27, 2017, https://www.livekindly.co/googles-executive-chairman-predicts-vegan-revolution-coming/.

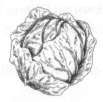

SUGGESTED RESOURCES

Books for kids:

And Here's to You! by David Elliott (Candlewick Press, 2009)

Benny Brontosaurus Goes to a Party by L. Farnsworth (SK Publishing, 2005)

Caterpillar Dreams by Clive McFarland (HarperCollins, 2017)

Charlotte's Web by E. B. White (Harper and Brothers, 2006)

Dave Loves Chickens by Carlos Patiño (Vegan Publishers LLC, 2013)

Does a Kangaroo Have a Mother, Too? by Eric Carle (HarperCollins, 2005)

Eating the Alphabet by Lois Ehlert (Harcourt Brace and Company, 1996)

The Forgotten Rabbit by Nancy Furstinger (The Gryphon Press, 2014)

Jasper's Story: Saving Moon Bears by Jill Robinson (Sleeping Bear Press, 2013)

Lena of Vegitopia and the Mystery of the Missing Animals: A Vegan Fairy Tale by Sybil Severin (Vegan Publishers, 2014)

Libby Finds Vegan Sanctuary by Julia Feliz Brueck (Vegan Publishers, 2016)

Make Way for Ducklings by Robert McCloskey (Puffin Books, reprinted 1999)

The One and Only Ivan by Katherine Applegate (HarperCollins, 2015)

Our Farm: By the Animals of Farm Sanctuary by Maya Gottfried (Knopf Books for Young Readers, 2010)

Piggy and Dad Go Fishing by David Martin (Scholastic, 2006)

Rah, Rah, Radishes! and *Go, Go, Grapes!* by April Pulley Sayre (Little Simon, 2014 and 2016 respectively)

Steven the Vegan by Dan Bodenstein (Totem Tales Publishing, 2012)

That's Why We Don't Eat Animals by Ruby Roth (North Atlantic Books, 2012)

'Twas the Night Before Thanksgiving by Dav Pilkey (Scholastic Paperbacks, 2004)

Vegan Is Love by Ruby Roth (North Atlantic Books, 2012)

Waiting for Wings by Lois Ehlert (HMH Books for Young Readers; first edition, 2001)

We're Vegan by Anna Bean (CreateSpace Independent Publishing Platform, 2013)

When the World Is Dreaming by Rita Gray (HMH Books for Young Readers, 2016)

Yertle the Turtle by Dr. Seuss (Random House, 2013)

Books for young adults and parents:

Above All, Be Kind: Raising a Humane Child in Challenging Times by Zoe Weil (New Society Publishers, 2003)

Becoming Vegan by Brenda Davis and Vesanto Melina (Book Pub Co., 2014)

The China Study by Dr. T. Colin Campbell (BenBella Books, 2006)

The Everything Vegan Pregnancy Book by Reed Mangels (Everything, 2011)

Farm Sanctuary: Changing Hearts and Minds About Animals and Food by Gene Baur (Touchstone, 2008)

The Great Life Cookbook by Priscilla Timberlake and Lewis Freedman (Coddington Valley Pub, 2013)

Help! There's a Vegan Coming for Dinner! by Karen Jennings (Art and Soul Interiors, 2016)

The Kind Mama: A Simple Guide to Supercharged Fertility, a Radiant Pregnancy, a Sweeter Birth, and a Healthier, More Beautiful Beginning by Alicia Silverstone (Rodale Books, 2014)

Living the Farm Sanctuary Life: The Ultimate Guide to Eating Mindfully, Living Longer, and Feeling Better Every Day, by Gene Baur (Touchstone, 2015)

Plant-Powered Families by Dreena Burton (BenBella Books, 2015)

Mercy For Animals: One Man's Quest to Inspire Compassion and Improve the Lives of Farm Animals by Nathan Runkle (Avery, 2018)

Mind If I Order the Cheeseburger? by Sherry F. Colb (Lantern Books, 2013)

Raising Vegan Children in a Non-Vegan World: A Complete Guide for Parents by Erin Pavlina (VegFamily.com, 2003)

The Skeptical Vegan by Eric C. Lindstrom (Skyhorse Publishing, 2017)

Skinny Bitch Bun in the Oven by Rory Freedman and Kim Barnouin (Running Press, 2008)

The 30-Day Vegan Challenge by Colleen Patrick-Goudreau (Roundtree Press, 2017)

Vegan for Her by Virginia Messina and JL Fields (Da Capo Lifelong Books, 2013)

The Vegan Pregnancy Survival Guide by Sayward Rebhal (Herbivore Books, 2011)

We Animals by Jo Anne McArthur (Lantern Books, 2017)

Films for young adults and parents:

Blackfish (CNN, 2013)

Earthlings (Nation Earth, 2005)

Forks Over Knives (Monica Beach Media, 2013)

Super Size Me (The Con, 2004)

What the Health (A.U.M. Films & Media, 2017)